THE SWITCH

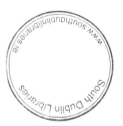

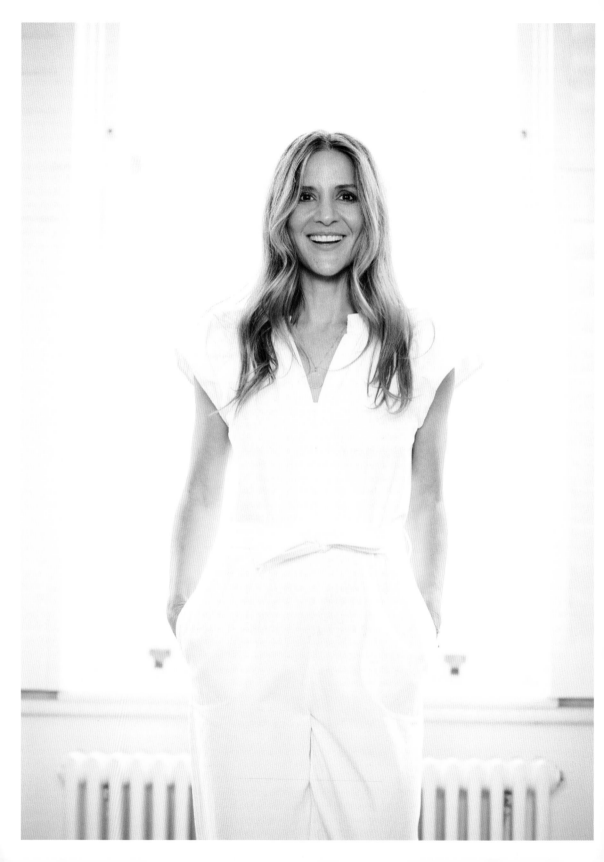

THE
SWITCH

—

THE SECRET
TO OVERCOMING THE
PRESSURES OF PERFECTION
AND FINDING HEALTH
AND HAPPINESS

—

AMANDA BYRAM

GILL BOOKS

Gill Books

Hume Avenue

Park West

Dublin 12

www.gillbooks.ie

Gill Books is an imprint of M.H. Gill and Co.

978 07171 89366

Lifestyle photography by **Ray Burmiston** (pp. ii, 18-19, 20, 28, 48, 56, 67, 76, 80, 89, 107, 120, 128-129, 152, 170, 194, 204, 228, 244) and **Julian Okines** (pp. viii-ix, x, 10, 37, 46-47, 62, 70-71, 72, 78-79, 98, 110-111, 112, 130, 138, 162-163, 164, 173, 176-177, 178, 184, 189, 192-193, 202-203, 212, 274)

Make-up and hair by Sally O'Neill

Styling by Annabel Kierman

Food photography by Leo Byrne

Food styling by Charlotte O'Connell

Copy-edited by Susan McKeever

Proofread by Jane Rogers

Printed and bound in Italy by Printer Trento

This book is typeset in 11pt on 13pt Futura Book.

The paper used in this book comes from the wood pulp of managed forests. For every tree felled, at least one tree is planted, thereby renewing natural resources.

5 4 3 2 1

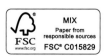

CONTENTS

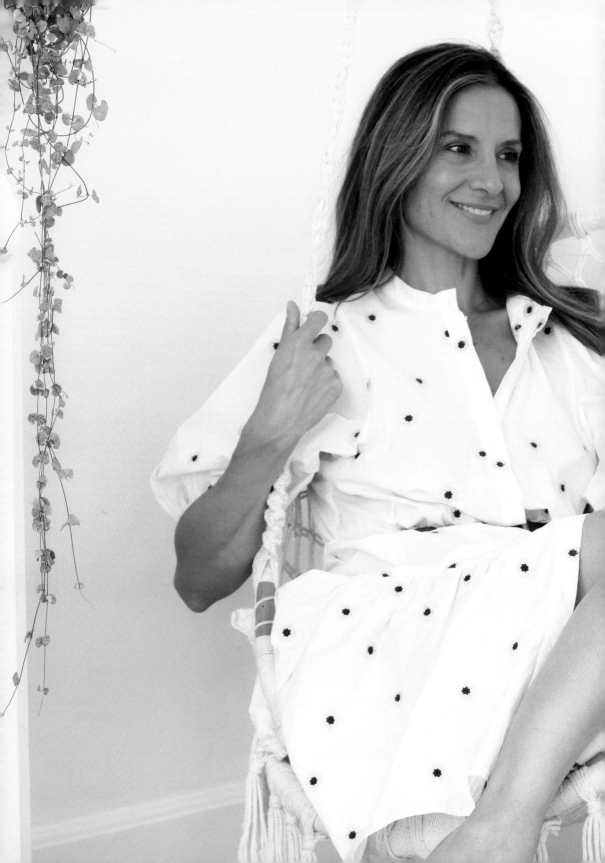

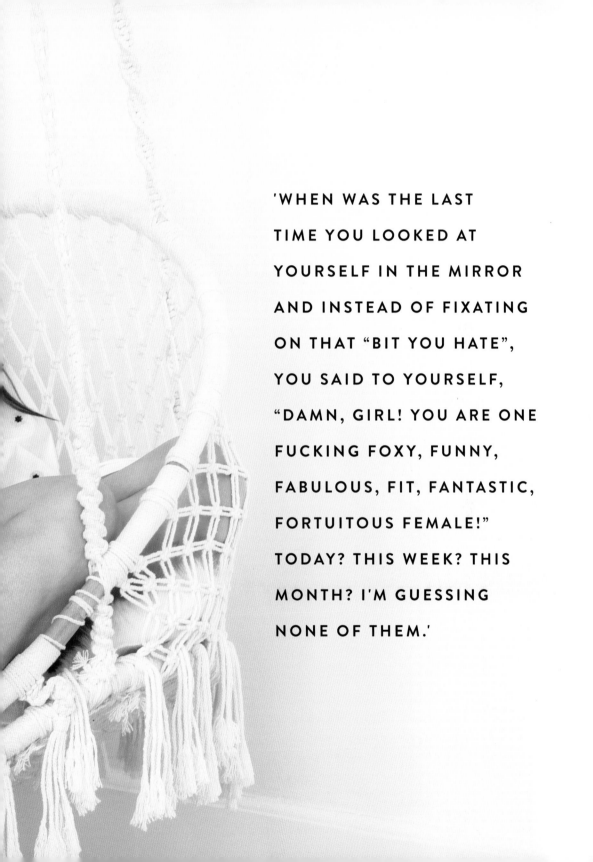

'WHEN WAS THE LAST
TIME YOU LOOKED AT
YOURSELF IN THE MIRROR
AND INSTEAD OF FIXATING
ON THAT "BIT YOU HATE",
YOU SAID TO YOURSELF,
"DAMN, GIRL! YOU ARE ONE
FUCKING FOXY, FUNNY,
FABULOUS, FIT, FANTASTIC,
FORTUITOUS FEMALE!"
TODAY? THIS WEEK? THIS
MONTH? I'M GUESSING
NONE OF THEM.'

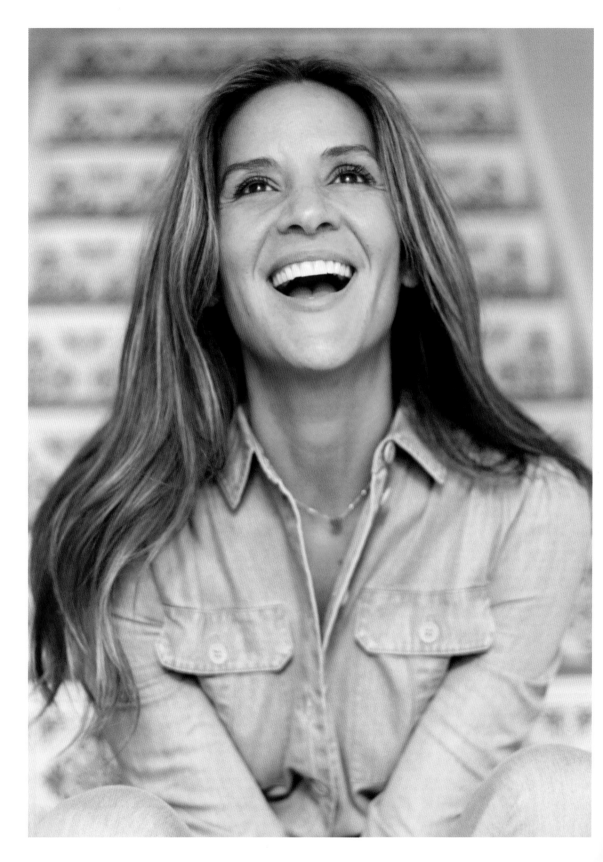

INTRODUCTION

FOR MOST OF my adult life I have been in the public eye – first as a model, and then as a TV presenter. Of course, an occupational hazard of being 'famous' (whatever the hell that means) is that you expose yourself to criticism from all angles, from tabloid takedowns to Twitter trolls. It used to hurt, so over the years I learned to protect myself by tuning it out. After all, opinions are like bumholes; everybody has one and they are mostly full of shit. However, despite my feisty approach, there was one critical voice who was bitch supreme and whom I could neither silence nor ignore. She was hypercritical, super-mean and relentless in reminding me where I was going wrong. She would set impossibly high standards in every aspect of my life and her favourite topic of criticism was invariably my food, my figure and my fitness. The worst part was that the critic was not a gossip journalist, a catty colleague or an online bully: it was me.

This voice would drive me to decades of desperate dieting and self-imposed misery. Having spoken to a lot of women from all walks of life, I now know that I am not alone in falling victim to this ruthless predator ... and once those claws take hold, it can be very hard to break free. For example, when was the last time you celebrated how truly amazing you are? When was the last time you looked at yourself in the mirror and instead of fixating on that 'bit you hate', you said to yourself, '*Damn, girl! You are one fucking foxy, funny, fabulous, fit, fantastic, fortuitous female!*' Today? This week? This month? I'm guessing none of them.

The sad truth is that most of us don't recognise our brilliance on a day-to-day basis and we haven't done so for a long while. We go through life focusing on our 'figure failures' and on the way we 'should' look or on the things we 'should' do. Of course, it is good to have aspirations, and being healthy is key to quality and quantity of life, so let's enjoy it along the way. How many of life's positive moments have to go unnoticed because we are too busy focusing on the negatives? How many times have you deprived yourself, only to look back and realise how awesome you actually looked and then think, 'Oh fuck, now I don't look like that anymore so I will just deprive myself again,' only to look back in another year and realise exactly the same thing ... you looked awesome! How many of our own sunny skies need to be darkened by clouds of our own making before we wake up and discover that so much of the shit we worry about is just not important?

We ignore our successes – and by successes, I don't mean climbing Mount Everest, winning Olympic medals or inventing the cure for the common cold. I mean the micro-wins we all achieve on a daily basis that enrich our lives and the lives of those around us, such as getting the kids off to school, completing a to-do list, making someone smile or taking time to get outside when you would rather slouch on the couch instead.

Even when we do spot these tiny wins, instead of celebrating them to the fullest, we perceive them as unworthy when compared to society's unrealistic portrayals of perfection. Particularly as women, we have become so accustomed to comparing ourselves we think we are letting everyone down unless we are J.Lo in the gym, Nigella in the kitchen, Oprah in the boardroom and Angelina in the nursery.

You might say, 'So am I meant to give myself a gold star like a little kid every time I take the stairs instead of the lift or give up my seat on the bus for an elderly passenger?' Well, would that be so bad? Would it be so bad if we started treating ourselves with the level of kindness and encouragement we might offer a child?

I remember being rewarded for even the tiniest of triumphs and smallest acts of kindness when I was a little girl growing up in Ireland. I was constantly praised and told how valuable I was ... how thoughtful I was ... how unique I was ... and it felt *really* good. Then somehow, as childhood faded, around the time of my sweet sixteen (or in my case sugar-free-sweetener sixteen) to pretty much my fortieth birthday, I allowed a more critical voice to speak up on my behalf and instead of championing my uniqueness, I started punishing myself for it. I listened to this voice and obeyed her every command as she mercilessly fixated on my figure. In time, and as a part of my healing process, I would come to call this voice out, name it, and give it an identity. I will get to this in more detail later.

The sacrifices I made during my never-ending journey for physical perfection seemed entirely justifiable even when the path took me to some seriously dark places riddled with twisty side-roads of confusion, rocky inclines of hunger, deep potholes of despair, mountains of grumpy moments and gloomy caves filled with fear, anxiety and general unhappiness. Worse still, I was oblivious to it all, which meant I wasn't even learning good lessons from bad decisions. Before I knew it, this narrative was dominating every daily decision. Fitness, fatness and everything in between had become an obsession.

Thinking back, it all seems uncharacteristic for me because, on the whole, I was a pretty well-rounded-has-her-shit-together type of girl. I was smart, well-liked outside my home and well-loved inside it. I enjoyed school and, later, art college, even though I secretly harboured aspirations of seeing my name in lights in Hollywood and marrying the Karate Kid (was it just me?). Along the way, I instinctively visualised my dreams and for the most part, they came true. After a short but fruitful career as a model, I co-anchored Ireland's first morning show, *Ireland AM*, which led to a move to London to host *The Big Breakfast* on Channel 4. Soon after, my visualised move to LA became a reality and I fronted various hit shows on Fox, which were seen by millions across the US. Almost a decade after I first drove up Sunset Boulevard, I moved back to the UK where, among other shows, I hosted several seasons of *Total Wipeout* on the BBC.

Over the years, I have expanded my professional portfolio to include not only TV presenter but also author, public speaker and brand owner. Although, full disclosure, I didn't marry the Karate Kid. The closest I came was dating a guy from New Jersey who had a black belt in karate … same-same.

With so many professional victories, I learned to trust my gut and listen to the voice inside my head that was supposedly serving me so well. However, achieving milestone after milestone so quickly meant that I didn't have time to assess whether I was succeeding *because* of this increasingly loud voice or *in spite* of it. In other words, I was beginning to convince myself that skinny = success and that if I looked exactly the way I wanted to, the rest would fall into place both personally and professionally. Forget Happy Ever After, the fairy-tale ending I was chasing was more like Skinny Ever After and I would do anything it took to get it.

THE DAWN OF THE SKINNY OBSESSION

—

It's hard to pinpoint exactly when this destructive voice uttered its first words. I suppose a pivotal moment was when I was 15, hanging out in my bedroom with my BFF. I distinctly recall us lying on my bed looking up at a poster of Morten Harket from A-ha and discussing, without any irony, ways we could get him to attend my upcoming birthday party (a girl can dream, right?). I was wearing my classic eighties uniform of cycling shorts and a Pepe Method T-shirt, and my gal pal innocently remarked on some 'fat' popping out of my shorts. While there was absolutely no malice intended in her comment, I do remember a switch flicking in my 15-year-old brain that perhaps started the long, exhausting, unromantic and abusive relationship I had with my body. It would take decades before I was able to flick the switch back to having a positive body image.

QUICK-FIX DIETS

The nineties didn't help because it was during this decade that my nemesis emerged – the quick-fix diet. Ever since they came into fashion, these diets have stuck to our psyches like non-fat-low-carb glue. I sought out and tried every quick-fix and deprivation diet that ever existed. I tried the cabbage soup diet, the grapefruit diet, the tomato and egg diet, the celery diet, the master cleanse, the Atkins diet, juice-fast diets, fat-free diets, full-fat and low-carb diets, high-protein, ketone, low-sugar diets, the 'we-don't-have-a-name-for-this-diet-yet-but-let's-tell-people-to-chew-air-and-call-it-the-Celebrity-Air-Diet' diet. You name it, I tried it.

At one stage, I spent an entire year consuming nothing but peaches, popcorn and SlimFast shakes every day. Needless to say, the lack of nutrition I was taking in that year was utterly ridiculous and I am amazed I survived without any lasting damage.

At that time my dietary advice was coming from the pages of daily newspapers and monthly magazines, and in a perverse twist of fate I was now beginning to feature in those very same magazines as I kicked off a career in modelling. In my mind, being on the pages of the magazines I had looked up to was justifying my dietary decisions as I unwittingly perpetuated the myth that 'thin is in' and skinny-at-all-costs was worth it.

Talk about the blind leading the blind.

My diet obsession gleefully linked my arm and accompanied me into my mid-twenties as my TV years came knocking. Although I ate healthy amounts of food, the food I was eating was not so healthy and it didn't go unnoticed. In fact, I have a caricature that the team at *Ireland AM* made for me when I left. The picture is of me, sitting in my host chair, with my hand in a box of Special K and a pot of black coffee beside me because, well, I was known to drink black coffee and graze on Special K all day.

It was around this time that the Atkins diet became a thing. For those of you unfamiliar with Atkins, it kicks off with a 'protein only' phase that is supposed to last for two weeks – mine lasted for almost three years. During that time neither a fruit nor a vegetable passed my lips. It was a time of high protein, low fibre, no carbs and, frankly, a lot of flatulence. Needless to say, I felt like shit. I was miserable and so was my body.

I managed to dabble professionally in diets for the best part of the next 15 years – if dieting had employees of the month, I would most certainly have dozens of framed certificates. Not something to be proud of. I found myself constantly going through a cycle that never seemed to end: I would feel 'fat' or just not quite as thin as I would like, read about a new diet, embark on it, mostly successfully, until I became utterly exhausted. With the exhaustion came capitulation and from time to time, the seal would break on my strict yet misguided eating practices. I would binge furiously on any sweet and/or chocolatey treat I could get my hands on but rather than making me feel better, it would make me feel worse. The thrill of the bad behaviour was always fleeting and would, of course, be followed by the obligatory period of guilt and self-flagellation. Worse still, the deprivation had confused my metabolism and any attempt to return to 'normal' eating patterns was met with weight gain as my body fought to store every calorie in preparation for the next period of starvation. Oh, and speaking of periods, I didn't menstruate for a whole year in my late teens because of extreme dieting and excessive exercise. Newsflash: The body is carefully monitoring your energy balance at all times to make sure it's in safe enough hands to make a baby. If you are reckless with your energy intake, your reproductive functions can often shut up shop and wait until an energy balance has resumed before opening back up.

I had become so caught up in the vicious circle of dieting and body image that I was destroying not just my metabolism (see p. 22) but also my self-worth and mental health. It was time to break free. Time to free myself from this abusive relationship with the negative voices in my head. I look back now at my younger self with a sense of sadness that with some better (or indeed any) guidance and education, I could have been physically healthy and, more important, mentally healthy as well.

Quick-fix diets were not the only addiction I was prey to – I was completely obsessed with exercise. Most days the first thought that entered my mind when I woke up would be, 'How am I going to get my exercise fix in?' Every day without fail, I would either head to the gym to lift weights or dive into a class for a blast of cardio. Some days I would do both. Looking back on my waking thoughts at that time, it was not excitement or pleasure I felt, more like anxiety.

I was training like an athlete would in the run-up to a competition, but the big day never came, because this was my whole life. As soon as I opened my eyes I would feel a sense of dread and stress, knowing that I had to make time for a workout, no matter what. Sometimes I'd set the alarm for 5 a.m., just to get in a quick run around the block before work. On one occasion when I was working on location, I had to set an alarm for 4 a.m., just to do some laps around the field and step-ups on the picnic benches. All of that would have been perfectly fine if I had wanted to do those sessions, but of course, I did not. I pushed myself to do them for fear of gaining weight, for fear that I would feel anxious and guilty during the day had I not had my 'fix'.

Exercise is wonderful and can make you feel ecstatic and will keep you healthy; it only becomes a problem when your mind starts to tell you that you must do something for fear of an irrational outcome. It then becomes an unhealthy obsession that rules your life, every single day.

SO HOW DID I DO IT?

—

Even though when the penny dropped it literally felt like a light switching on in my mind, it was not one single revelation that led to my emergence from the fog of addiction. It was a combination of realisations that built up over time to tip the scales. Once the switch had flipped, I had to do some work to replace old habits with new ones and retrain my brain back to sane:

- First, I educated myself about the science of how our bodies work and why the relationship between brain and body is so important.
- I learned how to eat well, exercise well and rest well as a sign of respect for the body I had finally learned to love.
- I learned that you *can* have a beautiful body without doing ugly things to yourself.
- Most of all, I learned that until I loved myself internally, no amount of external changes would matter.

A welcome side-effect of being happy and living healthily is that your body naturally sheds excess flab, your muscles tone up, your metabolism speeds up, your sleep improves and your energy levels go through the roof … #Winning.

As time went on, I developed more ways to quieten my mind from the maddening noise of negative thoughts. Now I possess a bag of tricks that I can pull out and use whenever I need to replace that noise with either a calming silence or gentle words of encouragement, and over the last few years I have been sharing these tricks with other women and found that they make a positive difference in their lives as well.

MY DISCLAIMER

What I cannot do is promise you that reading this book will solve all life's problems. In fact, let me get this disclaimer out of the way: buying this book alone will not make you healthy, happy, successful or more loved. The words you read are not magic spells, which upon uttering will transform you into a fairytale princess and make all your wildest dreams come true. If you bought this book expecting the aforementioned promise then I suspect that maybe you have been spending a lot of time and money buying self-help books assuming the author will do all the heavy lifting simply because you paid the money. Well from now on lady pants, let's agree on one thing: self-help books have the words 'self' and 'help' in them, which means it is up to you to HELP yourSELF.

Disclaimer aside, what I CAN promise you is that this book will be the nudge, the helping hand, the push up the bum, the words you needed to hear, the catalyst, The

Switch for you to achieve your goals all by yourself. Only YOU can promise to commit to being a version of yourself who has the imagination to envisage a journey and the guts to take the first step.

In the nineties sci-fi film *The Matrix*, Morpheus stands before Neo and asks him to either pick the red pill and carry on like nothing had happened, or swallow the blue pill and go on an adventure into the unknown. Well, this is your blue pill moment. If you are ready to go on a journey of self-discovery, self-assessment and self-discipline, then I'll be right by your side. If you are not ready, then no amount of persuading, pleading or punishing will make a difference.

And know this, unless you make The Switch in yourself, do not expect anything else in your life to fall into place. An old saying goes, 'When you get off the plane to paradise, the first person you meet is yourself.' That means that if you are expecting happiness to come along and give you a big slobbering kiss, you're missing the point. So stop wasting your life waiting for it to arrive on your doorstep and stop thinking that happiness is a destination. It's not. It's a state of mind that you simply have to find within yourself.

WHEN DO I MAKE THE SWITCH?

—

There is no bad time to make The Switch. You might be in your twenties and burning the candle at both ends, holding down a career and a solid party diary. You could be in your thirties, apparently 'healthy' yet slightly stressed and obsessed with clean eating. You could be in your forties or fifties and frantically trying to manage a career with kids pulling out of your sprog-soiled activewear or sandwiched between teens and ailing parents. Or you could be older, and want to make the most of your autumn years. Adopting this knowledge at ANY age is the key to the permanent change to be your best self.

Similarly, it doesn't matter if you are a size 8 or a size 18 – if you are fundamentally unable to live comfortably in your own skin, no physical changes will make you any happier. It took me 30 long years of making mistakes, accumulating knowledge, assimilating it, challenging the facts then making more of the same mistakes, until I learned enough to make The Switch and arrive at a place of peace.

So, I stand before you as a woman in her mid-forties wearing her heart on her sleeve, hoping to impart a little knowledge that could potentially save you years of hanger, confusion and anxiety by making the same mistakes I did. Together let's peel away the layers of lies and myths peddled by the media. Let's take the overwhelming heap of contradictory information and strip it back to basics. With a little bit of know-how, you can lose weight and get into shape the healthy way by taking back control of your relationship with food, your body and, most important, your mind.

DIET IS A DIRTY WORD

—

OK, let's get this bombshell well and truly exploded. DIETS. DON'T. WORK. They don't work philosophically, they don't work psychologically and they don't work physiologically. Not one bit. Never. No exceptions. Ever. Sure, you might have had weight-loss results with diets and define that as 'success', but know this: if your barometer for winning is based on the little numbers on those dreaded scales, then you are approaching this from the wrong angle because (and I'll say it again) diets don't work.

The first reason why 'diets' don't work is a question of linguistics. Somewhere along the way, this tiny, innocent and innocuous word has been sabotaged and changed from an accurate and matter-of-fact description of our daily eating habits into an emotionally charged and dangerous obsession that haunts our mealtimes. In short, we started out with Gizmo, didn't follow the rules and ended up with a fucking Gremlin.

Worse still, none of us noticed that the change was happening and when we did notice, we didn't see it as a problem. It's a lot like Sandra Dee's makeover in *Grease* – when you actually think about it, she went from being a strong, smart and independent woman into a leather-clad, cigarette-smoking, man-pleasing bimbo without any of us batting a heavily mascaraed eyelid. What she should have been singing was, 'Yeah, you're the one that I want, Danny, but I'm not going to dumb myself down and completely change my entire identity for you!'

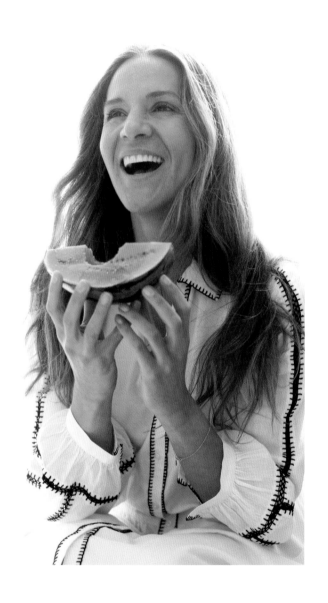

Anyway, I digress. If you are in the mood to get literal, the dictionary definition of the word 'diet' is 'how we typically or habitually eat', meaning a diet is not something you *do*, it's something you *have*. For those of us who remember primary school grammar lessons, the word 'diet' should really be treated as a noun rather than a verb. However, marketing execs, magazines and advertisers created an entire industry around 'dieting', making it the most overused and abused word in the world of health, food and nutrition. Nowadays, rather than having a good diet, we chase after the belief that going on a diet will fix our reckless food choices and help us get to where we need to be just in time for that holiday, wedding or school reunion.

I cannot stress this enough: *having* a good diet and *being* on a diet are two completely different things. One is the path to a well-balanced, healthy and happy existence; the other is a fast-track, one-way ticket to Crazytown where the streets are paved with guilt, shame, cravings, hunger and feelings of inadequacy.

Furthermore, the idea that 'one diet fits all' is absolutely and ridiculously ludicrous. You are unique in every way, right down to the way in which your body digests and processes nutrients. For example, some of us carry a gene that processes coffee more quickly, some of us deal with sugar more efficiently, some of us may be lactose intolerant and others may have a system that can burn calories much faster than others.

It is important that you take charge of your own body. No one knows your body, or how it feels, better than you do. That is why it is crucial that you listen to the language your body is speaking – translating what it is telling you will help you to develop a healthy relationship with food.

So let's make a pledge right here and now to reject the metastasised definition of the artist formerly known as Diet and go back to the way it used to be before it was a dirty word. To make things easier, let's call going on a diet a quick-fix diet (QFD) or a deprivation diet (DD) and by calling them out, we can see them for what they really are. Oh, and bonus points ... you've just unwittingly engaged in a little Neuro-Linguistic Programming (NLP) which we'll get on to in more depth later (see page 84).

At this point the QFD lovers among you might be fighting the urge to hastily thumb forward through the pages to get to the 'lose weight at the speed of light' section. And when you don't find it, beads of sweat might begin to form on your brow, as you flip frantically through the book to see where the page is that explains how you can 'eat this celery that only grows in the deepest, darkest region of Peru, and you will be skinny'. And when you don't find that, you might go to your purse to see if you kept the receipt for this book, and take it back in exchange for the *Atkins Meets Master Cleanse Diet Extravaganza Bumper Edition*.

STOP! This book isn't about quick fixes, and unless you get your mind in shape, your body is always going to struggle to keep up. I won't lie; there will be times during this process when you'll be mentally exhausted. That's OK. Big changes take time and if you take on too much at once, neglect will inevitably set in and failure will follow. It is important to remember to be patient. As the philosopher Nietzsche famously said: 'He who would learn to fly one day must first learn to stand and walk and run and climb and dance; one cannot fly into flying.'

Things do not happen immediately – they happen slowly and surely. Why do you think so many women try and fail to lose weight or to look and feel their best? Because when we set our expectations too high, impatience is sure to follow. We live in a society where everything is available right now. And in turn, this fuels our desire and hunger to have everything we want readily available. We want the quick-fix diet, speedy slimming pills and instant abs. We want skin that looks 20 years younger in 10 minutes. We want disposable content and we want it faster and faster, so much so that Netflix and digital platforms are struggling to keep up. Whatever happened to watching one episode of your show ... on the telly ... per week? Nowadays, we want to binge-consume and then move on. It is important to stay still in the moment, acknowledge what's happening and how you want to rectify it. We have been told by society that if we want to lose weight quickly, the only way to get there is to severely deprive ourselves, restrict calories and even cut out certain food groups altogether. This just isn't the case and is not the key to long-lasting health and happiness.

Magazines and the media hold a lot of responsibility for this sad state of affairs, often making bold proclamations that they care about our wellbeing, all the while using visuals that are breaking us down both physically and mentally. It breaks my heart when I see cover after cover of retouched 'perfection' and what they perceive to be a 'perfect size 8'. Equally maddening are the headlines that make promises as to how we can 'lose 7lb in 7 days', or how we can achieve that 'beach body just in time for summer'. It creates so much confusion.

And I'm not blameless in that. I readily admit that there have been times when I have been on the wrong side of the fence and images of me in magazines when I was younger perpetuated a myth of wellbeing through my own extreme dieting. Well, I am here now to atone by shining a light on how to fix the problem. Together we can stop buying into the lies, subscribing to the non-truths and find some equanimity by working towards true health and genuine happiness. And on the subject of blame ...

YOU ARE NOT TO BLAME

—

If you are feeling confused, anxious and frustrated about your relationship with food and the unattainable quest for physical perfection, please know that you are not to blame for thinking this way, so unburden yourself now of any guilt and shame.

Sailing the shiny seas of consumerism can be dangerous because lurking in the depths are big, scary, capitalist sharks ready to gobble us up if we aren't careful. While we are all the captain of our own ship, the water is often clouded by clever advertising and mixed messaging. That means images of perfection on one side and endless opportunities for 'consequence-free calorie consumption' on the other. Make no mistake, if you dive right in, these 'sharks' will be waiting, ready to feast.

So be mindful, most of all when food is involved. When you walk into a supermarket, what is the first aroma that greets you? It's the smell of freshly baked bread and croissants – and that is no coincidence. Supermarkets spend millions on psychological research every year in order to trick you into a sneaky consumer journey that begins with baked goods and ends with an impulse-buy chocolate bar at the checkout. Along the way, the shelves are stacked with low-calorie, low-fat, high-protein and no-added-sugar packaging that is designed to lure us in, like the Child Catcher's carriage from *Chitty Chitty Bang Bang*. Thus, without you even knowing it, your local supermarket has been subtly sparking the parts of your brain that trigger a symphony of different emotions, cravings and desires as you meander innocently through the aisles.

THE LABELLING LIE

Don't get me started on labelling. Labels are put on foods because it is against protocol to sell an item that has been produced, created or manufactured without telling us what's inside it. Food companies love a label because it allows them to jump on trends and, in doing so, disguise important information with shiny big claims.

Take a protein bar, for example. It can often contain a slew of unhealthy ingredients including stabilisers, preservatives and sugars, but because it contains just a small amount of protein, the brand can write 'HIGH PROTEIN' on the front and pass it off as healthy. Unless you are paying attention, you are likely to only see the words 'HIGH' and 'PROTEIN', completely bypassing the sugar content and the long list of other crap contained within. By the time you get to the checkout you have a trolley full of foods you didn't intend to buy, and a head full of anxiety.

THE DRIVE TO CONSUME SADS

And it doesn't end in the supermarket. Now think of a Friday night trip to the cinema to watch the latest Marvel movie. Yes, it's great fun and we all enjoy gazing up at superheroes and their perfectly sculpted silhouettes saving the day on the silver screen, but what happens when you look down? Most likely, you'll see a large popcorn and Diet Coke combo in your lap that costs pennies to produce, yet is sold for much, much more. The plot thickens ... could this perhaps be the cinema's *real* business model and why the ticket stand is also the snack counter?

By the time the credits have rolled and the movie is over, the image of Hollywood perfection remains in your mind but there's something else: a nagging feeling that you binged on chunks of sugary air and sugary water and that you definitely have to go on a diet come Monday morning.

Again, this is not your fault. You are caught in a tug of war between the conscious desire to look like a movie star and the unconscious need to cave in to cravings. And speaking of caves, remember that your brain originally evolved to deal with a very different, prehistoric environment where food, in particular sugar, was a rarity.

Today, that is completely different. Food is abundant but your brain still thinks it's dealing with life around the campfire. Worse still, everywhere we go, someone, somewhere, somehow is trying to get us to consume as much sugar, alcohol and drugs (or, as I call them, 'SADs' – see page 49) as is humanly possible. And this is no coincidence because there is so much money to be made from us, the unconscious consumers.

As well as trying to resist the urges of our cavewoman brains, we are also trying to unlearn the behaviours that we were unwittingly taught as children. Think of a Disney princess plastered on the side of a McDonald's Happy Meal. As little girls we were taught to idolise and aspire to be like these perfect beauties who enjoy fame, fortune and the love of a prince, while being encouraged to find 'happiness' in a box containing a burger, chips, a Coke and a toy of the aforementioned princess. Think again about the name for just a second and it is enough to make you scream: 'Happy Meal'. Newsflash: this meal will *not* make you happy! Whether we like it or not, everywhere we turn – from subliminal advertising to social media – we are being sold a lie. These lies and contradictions have understandably caused confusion, and that needs to change.

So what is to be done? There's no point in hoping that the food industry will grow a conscience – this is about as likely as your pet cat winning a Nobel prize for astrophysics. Let's instead attempt to take control back from a rigged system that relies on our desperation to look and feel a certain way and then sells us the short-term solution where we happily shove our hands into our pockets, take out our emotional pennies, and buy into those lies every day.

If we leave it up to someone else to fix us, we'll inevitably keep failing and coming back for more torture, again and again. Let's face it, if we were all 100 per cent healthy and happy, how would the sugar, tobacco, alcohol or indeed the pharmaceutical industries make their money? Our downfalls and confusion equate to their mansions in the Hamptons. Are you OK with that? I am not. Don't let the system fool you! Don't let the fuckers lead you round by the stomach because if you go into the big, bad world with your eyes closed and your mouth open you are going to make bad decisions that ultimately benefit a system that has been set up for you to fail.

Without mental health, physical health will be fleeting and will not lead to happiness. The data backs this up: according to the Mental Health Foundation, if we are unhappy with our bodies, it's likely that it will lead to an 'overall poorer quality of life, psychological distress and the risk of unhealthy eating behaviours and eating disorders'. Worse still, according to the BSAS (British Social Attitudes Survey), 'women's body satisfaction does not automatically improve as they move toward and into midlife, indeed, a 45-year-old woman is as likely to be as dissatisfied with her appearance as her 19-year-old daughter'.

The level of body image issues among women and young girls is at an all-time high – almost 90%. And here is the scariest part: when asked, many young women revealed that their mothers were responsible for passing on their own insecurities. So if ever there was a motivation to finally get your head straight, it's that the body image issues that have plagued you for decades are now looking to get their grubby paws on your daughter's psyche, and she will take that with her into *her* forties and beyond. So regardless of your age, let's get rid of our fixations with six packs, thigh gaps and skinny jeans.

In a nutshell, you just cannot achieve prime physical health without being mentally healthy, and vice versa. They are two sides of the same coin, and that coin is priceless. It is the currency to ultimate happiness. In order to *look* different you will need to *think* differently, then your mind and body can start to work in harmony rather than being in conflict with each other.

So let's educate ourselves as to WHY diets don't work for your body and cut through the bullshit with regard to what food actually is and does, and why we need it to not only survive but also thrive.

- Every morning, when you get out of bed, stand in front of a full-length mirror and give yourself some unconditional love: Say out loud three times, 'Damn, girl! You are one fucking foxy, funny, fabulous, fit, fantastic, fortuitous female!' The little wins are enough, you are good enough, and you deserve the happiness.

- Get yourself a calendar and some gold stars and start rewarding yourself every time you achieve a micro win. Don't trade them for anything; it is just a great way to remind yourself that life's little moments are worth celebrating and that the little things you do on a daily basis truly matter.

- Write your own bio and remember to include all the moments you are proud of! I found writing my career highlights for this chapter was a really useful way to review and celebrate the life successes I have enjoyed.

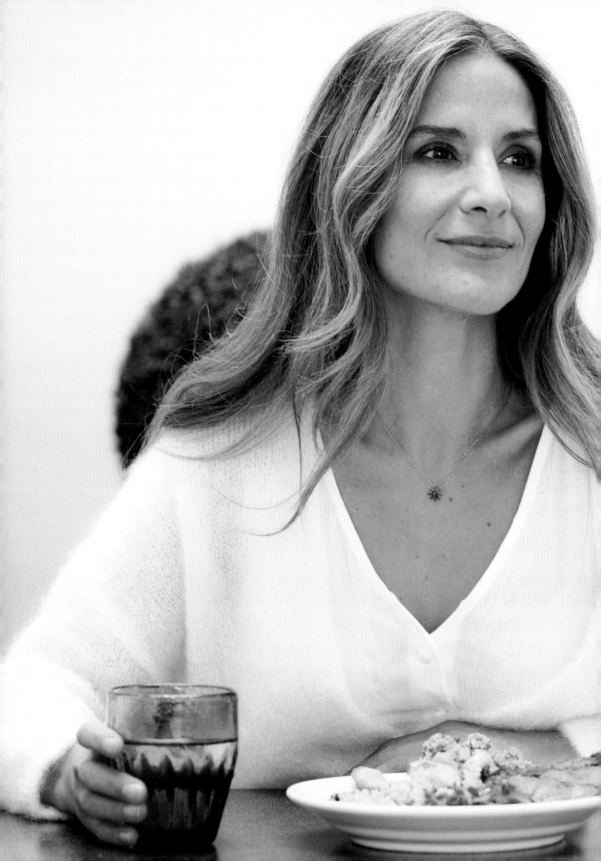

'YO-YO DIETING
CAN EASILY BECOME
ADDICTIVE, BOTH
PSYCHOLOGICALLY AND
PHYSICALLY, AND THE
FURTHER DOWN THE
RABBIT HOLE YOU GO,
THE MORE DANGEROUS
IT CAN BECOME.'

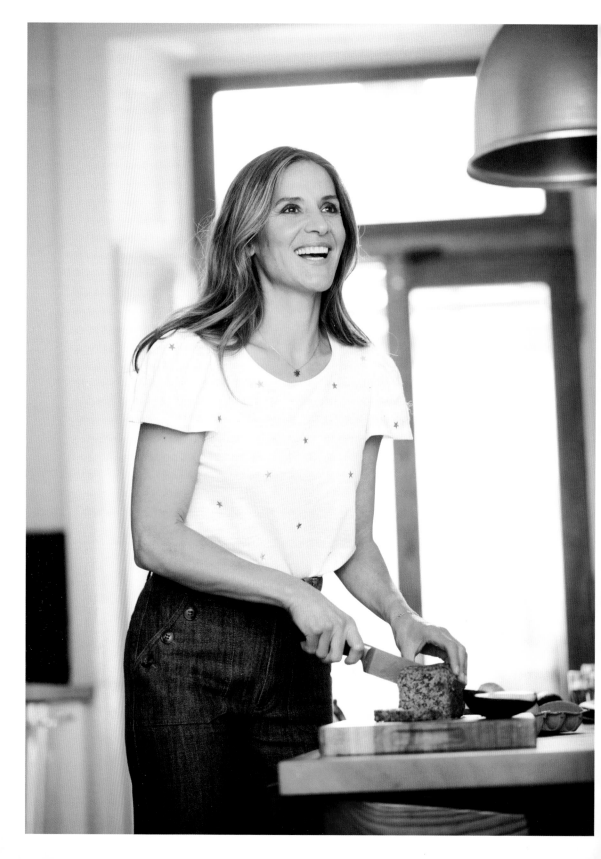

WHY
DIETS DON'T
WORK

THE MESSED UP THING about QFDs is that if you dabble in them enough they become addictive, not because they work, but because they don't work. Worse still, the yo-yoing can easily become addictive, both psychologically and physically, and the further down the rabbit hole you go, the more dangerous it can become. This is because with each new attempt to diet, your body adapts to deal with what it believes to be a crisis. And crisis it is, because over time the results can become catastrophic.

Tell me if this sounds familiar. You look in the mirror and don't like what you see. You just read about the 'Lose 10lb in 10 minutes' diet and so without a second thought, you grit your teeth and clamp your mouth shut ready to embark on a severely restrictive food intake.

At first, it works ... Hallelujah! There's a noticeable shift in weight (pretty logical given the deprivation – here's looking at you Mr Atkins). However, something else starts to happen. You are feeling significantly less energetic. You notice a dip in immunity. Your digestion is troublesome (yes I'm talking to you, Miss Farty-pants). To boot, the initial weight loss has plateaued, leaving you feeling frustrated, moody and turning green as you begin to grumble with increasing frequency, 'You won't like me when I'm hangry.'

Eventually it all becomes too much, and you abandon the QFD ship only to find that the weight you initially lost cascades back on, accompanied by a head full of mental anguish. You begin to curse the QFD and feel some sort of shame because you feel bad about your body and what you have just put it through. The chances are that you now blame *yourself* for this weight gain, telling yourself that you are not just fat, you are also stupid and incapable.

And here is where things get dangerous. Just like a junkie you begin to look for the next QFD or DD, to shift the weight you just gained. And so begins the vicious cycle and you end up in a maelstrom of deprivation, purge, binge, and repeat, until you ultimately crash and burn. All the while not understanding that from the start, you were never destined to succeed.

So why did it actually fail?

METABOLISM AND THE AFTERMATH

—

The answer is simple. QFDs and DDs fuck with your body's metabolic rate, which is the time it takes for your body to process your food, extract the nutrients, create some energy, and do all the things you need to do before getting rid of the waste (poo-poo and pee-pee alert).

Think of your metabolism like this: you are the boss of your body and part of being the boss means paying your worker the right salary. Pay her well and also give her bonuses every time she performs and you'll have an employee of the month, every month, for life.

In contrast, if you pay your employee below the minimum wage and expect her to work her ass off, then sorry, you are going to have an unhappy employee who will keep taking sick leave and be sluggish and asleep on the job.

And if you pay too much over a prolonged period, she might get lazy and be less inclined to work because she knows she will be able to keep herself in riches without lifting a finger.

If there is one thing your employee loves, it is a consistent salary. And ultimately YOU dictate the varied states of your metabolism, and whether your metabolism is fast, middle-of-the-range or slow, it is primarily adapting to the environment you create according to the nutrients you are feeding it.

- If you feed it well and exercise, you can afford to continue to eat well and perform well.
- If you feed it too much but do not exercise, you will begin to build calories and gain weight.
- If you do not feed it enough and expect to still be healthy, you will have to work hard to get it back in favour.

If only I had paid my employee a consistent wage I could have saved myself decades of deprivation and union strikes. It took me years to just unravel the simplicity of this mechanism of the body that I now honour, obey and respect.

After each new QFD your body finds it very difficult to settle again and starts to take pre-emptive measures. When you start eating 'normally', i.e. balanced amounts of macro and micronutrients (see page 27), your body panics and stockpiles food calories for energy; it knows that soon it may be starved and may need a reservoir of energy to carry out everyday tasks – in other words, to exist.

In short, when you adopt a restrictive diet, you are effectively starving yourself. Of course, your body doesn't know this starvation is self-imposed, so it responds in a few crucial ways to 'help' you get through it and survive. First, you'll experience an increase in appetite as your body calls out for nutrients (cravings, anyone?). If you ignore the appetite increase and continue to diet, your body starts to panic about when the next proper meal will come along, so it slows down your metabolism to ensure energy is spent more carefully. This translates as less pep for daily life and even shutting down non-essential processes (goodbye, periods). The result is a slow metabolism and a massive appetite. So, when you give in to the cravings (or stop your diet), you'll want to eat everything in sight and your body won't be able to process it properly. Long story short, you'll pile on the pounds and conclude the only way to solve the problem is to 'go on a diet'! As physically dangerous as this process is, what comes next is even scarier. Without understanding why, you'll start viewing food as the problem, not the dieting, and before long you'll be stuck in a cycle of disordered eating.

WHAT EVEN *IS* A CALORIE?

—

Right, let's talk about the 'C' word ... calories. For decades, calorie counting has restricted people's diets. And while the practice has brought misery and deprivation to most, it has brought relative success to others. The thing is, the success stories will most likely NOT have been as a result of some ingenious calorie theoretical chart, but simply from restricting highly calorific foods. In other words, could it be that the success of calorie counting is not actually due to the immaculate counting of calories, and rather down to the reduction in portion size? In which case, it's pretty obvious there will always be a modicum of success.

Even though maintaining a healthy weight should be as simple as balancing calories in with calories out, how do we know that the 'calorie' figures we are accustomed to on food labels are even accurate?

The idea of calories relating to nutrition came into being more than 100 years ago when their daddy, an American chemist called Wilbur Atwater, burned foods and measured the temperature of the heat they released. The change in temperature was an indication of the energy the food offered. Through a series of boring equations (sorry, Wilbur), he came up with a figure (measured in kilocalories, or kcal) for each food group. The formula that was created is the one we stick to today: protein has 4 kcal per gram; fat 9 kcal per gram; carbohydrate 4 kcal per gram and so on.

The reason I am mentioning the vague accuracy of calorie counting is this: first, Daddy Wilbur's equations were estimated, and burning food as a measure is massively over-simplifying things. And second, chemist Atwater didn't take into account things such as each person's individual response to the food type. There are so many factors that determine how food is digested, absorbed and used. Not to mention the variations in how food is cooked, stored and grown, or the fact that one would not ordinarily eat each food type by itself – most meals are a combination of carbohydrates, fats, proteins, etc. (see page 27). Since we humans do not live in a lab, nor are we walking bomb calorimeters (that carry out individual experiments on each food we consume), the variations of results are endless. Hence, the figures on a food label or package are estimates and can often be extremely different in reality.

Needless to say, in the hundred-plus years since Wilbur and his esteemed colleagues first suggested their method of measuring calories, we have come a long way in understanding how the body absorbs nutrients. My point is that calories are a hard thing to quantify, so tirelessly counting them may be more exhausting and counter-productive than you think. Also, if you're trusting what is reported on food labels you should be aware that they can overstate or understate the amount of calories in foods. This is plain and simply confusing and can also have health risks.

Also, remember that measuring calories out is just as tough as counting calories in. For example, when I do a workout, my iWatch tells me I have burned 200 calories. However, the effect of exercise can stay with you long after you have left the gym, so focusing on what you have burned will leave you with only part of the picture.

Yes, of course it is important to be mindful of the amounts of foods you eat that are higher in calories in general, because the simple equation of approximate calories in versus approximate calories out through exercise or normal daily activities will keep you at the same approximate weight. But it's also important not to focus too much on, or become obsessed with calories and calorie counting. This is when food becomes the enemy, and eating becomes a chore as opposed to a ceremonial occasion.

ENJOYING FOOD

—

It makes me sad to see the way that food has become weaponised in a war against our bodies. We've also seen the demonising of entire food groups like carbohydrates and fats – foods that are actually essential to a healthy, well-functioning metabolism.

Traditionally, food was eaten ceremonially and was at the centre of happy, convivial occasions when friends and families got together and enjoyed hearty, wholesome meals. This tradition is slowly dying, and many of us seem to have lost the joy of eating.

When you eat on the run, stress eat or shame eat, your body is in a natural state of distress: you're looking at the clock, panicking that you have to finish quickly and get back to work, or eating the food quickly before you notice the calorie content. This means you will most likely not be chewing your food properly, and are therefore missing out on a vital part of the digestive process by unlocking nutrients more efficiently. Mastering the art of mastication will also reduce the temptation to overeat, as your brain has more time to realise that your body is full.

Did you know that chewing also stimulates pleasurable neurotransmitters? This explains our enjoyment around eating food. Eating good food and eating it mindfully gives so many positive rewards because your body will receive the good nutrients, you will be fuller for longer and, more important, your body will not be in a state of stress or panic. Eat every meal with intention, and treat food as a gift to your body and not as an enemy.

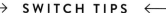

SWITCH TIPS

- Quit playing around with yo-yo dieting; it's like playing with fire for your metabolism. It's a risky game and one that doesn't usually pay off.

- Dieting will mess with your metabolism, resulting in weight gain and lifelong issues with how your body metabolises food in the future.

- Don't obsess over every calorie. Keep an eye on them if you do not want to over-consume, but remember it is so much more important to enjoy your food. Food is your friend, not your enemy; so pick your battles.

- Don't cut out food groups, don't deny yourself something if you really want it and don't stress about food – it's counter-productive.

- No one way of eating fits all, so listen to *your* body, not the body of your 'friend' on Instagram. What works for them may not work for you. Your body may not tolerate the same foods as them. Your body is unique, so do what it tells you to do.

- Enjoy your food; otherwise you might as well be eating cardboard or cotton wool. As a rule of thumb, try to be mindful every time you eat. Take a moment to close your eyes, or if not, then at least have a moment to take a deep breath before you take a bite. Chew your food properly, taste the flavour and feel the texture before swallowing.

FOOD GROUPS

—

We have established that the key is not to 'be' on a diet but to 'have' a good diet that keeps you energetic, nourished and alert. Further still, having a 'balanced' diet is consistent with long-term mental and physical health.

But what the fuck does a 'balanced' diet even mean? Some of us think it means 'no wine Monday to Friday and then I can test out half the wines in the off licence between 12 p.m. on a Saturday and midnight on a Sunday'. Others think it means 'carb-free during the week and an all-bets-off carb-fest on the weekends'. And some of us think that 'well-balanced' means 'a plate of spag bol in one hand, a burger in another, and see which one is heavier'.

Of course it is none of the above.

In fact the first two scenarios are classic examples of those old-fashioned binge–purge cycles that get our metabolisms into so much trouble.

'Balance' means knowing what is good for you and having a little bit of all of it. It's not about weighing it, bingeing it, purging it, hiding it or counting it. It is about letting your body decide when enough is enough and giving your body the benefit of the doubt. But before you can have balance it is important to understand *what* you are eating. And that starts with knowledge of food groups.

To be clear, a food group is not a bunch of people sitting in a circle discussing their favourite meals. Food groups consist of macros and micros, the macros being the big kahunas: protein, carbohydrates, fats and fibre. The micros consist of vitamins and minerals.

So let's digest (pun intended!) what each of these does and hence understand why we should *never* cut out any food group.

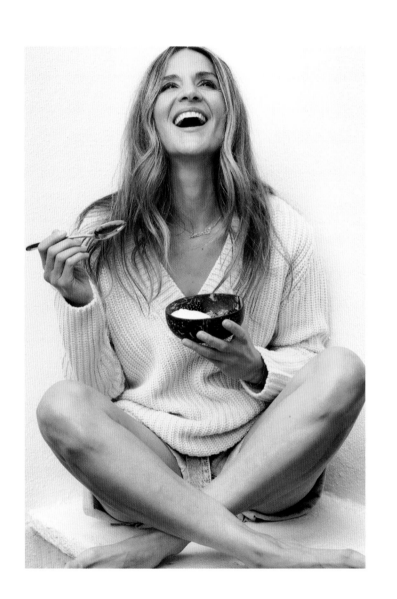

PROTEIN: THE BUILDING BLOCKS OF LIFE

—

Proteins are made up of amino acids, which are sort of like tiny Lego blocks. They are the building blocks of life. Some of these Lego blocks we can make in our body, others we have to get from food – hence these are called 'essential amino acids'.

When we eat protein, our bodies rearrange these Lego blocks to form hair, skin, bone, teeth and nails. In short, protein is vital for life and highlights how important it is to get good sources of protein in your daily diet. However, too much protein can be a bad thing and here's why.

A relatively active woman needs the equivalent of approximately 40–60g of protein in her diet every day. Now let's consider that a skinless chicken breast contains 54g of protein, which means that this one chicken breast contains enough protein for a healthy female body to do its daily thing. The amount we require increases the more active we are, yet even then consuming extra protein in protein shakes, protein bars, protein cereals or protein waters is entirely unnecessary, despite what the supplement industry would have you believe.

Now for the really scary part. Your body cannot store protein or use more protein than it needs, so any excess (if not used as energy) will be tough on your kidneys and excreted as urine (which means you are literally pissing your money away when you buy too many protein shakes) or ... (shock horror) the excess calories from eating too much protein could lead to weight gain over time.

If weeing excessively (with an extra pungent strong smell) rings a bell then perhaps you've had more than your fair share of protein. If that is the case, you have an increased risk of kidney damage and also unexplained weight gain.

Many people argue about the best sources of protein, and I believe that the key lies in the *quantity and quality* of the protein.

FISH: my personal favourites are salmon, prawns, scallops, cod and sea bass.

WHITE MEAT: turkey and chicken are great sources of animal protein, but always try to buy from a good source and make sure they're free-range.

RED MEAT: beef, lamb, and pork, grass-fed where possible to avoid steroids.

OTHERS: eggs, pulses (such as chickpeas and lentils), dairy, soya, grains and superfoods (such as spirulina and hemp).

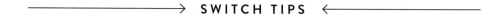

SWITCH TIPS

- Protein is the key to feeling fuller for longer and helps to rebuild your muscles after workouts.

- Too much protein can cause excess nitrogen in the body that needs to be excreted, and it can also lead to weight gain.

- Most foods contain some protein, so rotate your protein sources daily where possible.

- Don't get sucked into the protein-craze fads.

- If you're a meat eater, switch from red meat to white meat at least once a week, or switch all meat to fish.

- While we're on the subject of fish, switch fried, breaded or battered fish to grilled, steamed or stir-fried fish. Those coatings can be high in fat, salt and sugar.

- Go vegetarian or vegan twice a week by switching all your animal protein (including fish) to plant-based protein. You can include pulses such as beans, lentils, soya beans and alfalfa or soya-based products such as tofu or tempeh.

- Switch from low-fat dairy products, such as milk and yoghurt, to smaller amounts of full-fat versions. Low-fat products are pumped with extra sugar.

- Switch your morning oatmeal to other protein-rich grains that you can cook the same way as oats, such as barley flakes, spelt, cornmeal, kamut (an ancient grain), quinoa or buckwheat. It is easy to add nut butter and milk for a high-protein breakfast.

WHAT'S THE VEGAN DEAL?

—

Hands up if you grew up eating meat. Hands up if you grew up being told that meat and two veg is the best all-round meal. Hands up if you believe that vegans do not get enough protein to be strong. Hands up if you are a little bit confused about why vegetarians and vegans are still breathing and some even look fantastic.

Up until only a few years ago I would have put my hand up for all of the above. My belief was that eating animal protein was not just a necessity; I was made to believe that it held the key to a good training regime and was the secret to the perfect meal and the source of all vitamins essential to overall health.

Eating a plant based diet might seem counter-intuitive to those of us who grew up on a meat and two veg diet, but slowly and steadily we are learning about the reality of the effects of animal protein on our bodies. Even professional athletes have reported that going plant-based has turned them into gold medal-winning machines. But how can a vegan get enough protein to be strong? Surely without meat, there are not enough plants that could ever sustain this level of protein intake. Right?

Wrong.

The notion that we need an abundance of meat to perform well, or at high levels, is simply not true, and while there are some benefits to eating the flesh of animals (including to satisfy an individual's personal taste preference), there is a high probability that we have been sold a little bit of a meaty lie. Here's why.

Traditionally, the logic has been that meat contains every single amino acid (those 'Lego' blocks I mentioned earlier) your body could need. However, essential amino acids can also be found in an array of plant-based foods such as pulses, root vegetables and grains. After all, cows only eat grass and they are more stacked than Schwarzenegger! And get this, just one cup of lentils or a peanut butter sandwich, has about as much protein as 85 grams of meat or three large eggs! The quality of plant-based protein is *not* inferior, as some meat-eating storytellers would have you believe.

Therefore, if we eat a varied plant-based diet our bodies are clever enough to assimilate all the different amino acids we need to function normally and more. The added bonus is that a plant-based diet is lower in saturated fats (see page 39), kinder to the environment and also a little more ethical – meaning we can be healthier while having a clearer conscience.

At this stage some of you may be thinking, 'But what about vitamins in meat? Surely B12 is an important vitamin that is closely linked to meat eating?'

This is also a common misconception, because although B12 is found in animal protein, it is not because animals *make* it, but because they either consume it from the soil, which contains B12-producing bacteria, or they are supplemented with it. Therefore, a vegan is just as likely to get their B12 from a plant-based diet as a meat eater is to get it from their steak.

Unfortunately, the pesticides and antibiotics used in industrial farming are wiping our veggies clean of the bacteria that produces B12, so it is prudent for meat eaters, vegans or anyone on a plant-based diet to look at taking a B12 supplement because of the practices involved in industrial farming.

Overall, food choices are personal and whether you are a carnivore, vegan, vegetarian, pescatarian or flexitarian, it is important to be mindful of how you eat and what you eat because your daily dietary decisions will impact both the health of your body and that of our planet.

THE OTHER 'C' WORD: CARBOHYDRATES

—

So we get to the villain of the piece. A macronutrient so hated, feared and reviled that most dieters think the only way to get slim is to avoid it at all costs. I am of course speaking about the dreaded carbohydrate. However, the exact opposite is true because carbohydrates are essential for getting healthy, being healthy and staying healthy. Period. There, I said it.

The problem is that although you just read those words, I know that deep down you still believe carbs to be the bad guy. And that is understandable because the 'No carbs before Marbs' slogan, made famous by the British reality show *TOWIE*, is a pretty difficult one to shift. And like all myths that swirl about in the media and online, separating the fact from the fiction is the key to making mindful choices rather than simply swallowing the low-carb lies.

I spent years of my life as a 'carb avoider' and there were costs in almost every aspect of my life. I was always tired, I had constant brain fog, I was often irate, grumpy or argumentative and I experienced low libido (GAH!). Probably the biggest irony of carb dodging was that I did not have enough energy to enjoy exercise and so would frequently get annoyed with myself for underperforming. Subsequently I denied myself further carbs to compensate and the more I bought into the 'carbs are evil' story, the worse it got. I was trapped!

It was only when I decided to study nutrition that I learned the exact science behind carbohydrates and why we really do need them. Here is what I learned:

Carbohydrates are sugar molecules stitched together in varying lengths and can be categorised as either simple or complex. The longer the chain, the longer it takes for your body to break down the links and extract the energy.

SIMPLE CARBOHYDRATES

Simple carbohydrates are (obvious alert) single sugar molecules. So, by their very nature, they act quickly and give shorter bursts of energy in the body.

Let's say you eat 100 grams of sugar found in a bag of Percy Pig jellies. Your body will absorb the sugar very quickly and therefore give you an instant burst of energy. That energy will not last for long though, and you will soon come crashing down.

Examples of food that contain simple carbohydrates (sugar) are:

- Cakes (sponge, muffins and buns)
- Biscuits
- Sweets
- White bread
- White pasta
- White flour
- Alcohol
- Fruit juices
- Sauces (ketchup, BBQ sauce, spaghetti sauce)
- Flavoured yoghurts
- Breakfast cereals and shop-bought granola
- Low-fat foods
- Fizzy drinks (excluding sparkling water!)

COMPLEX CARBOHYDRATES

Complex carbohydrates are branch chains of sugar molecules; being complex, they take longer for the body to break down and process.

Have you ever had a tangled necklace? Of course you have! Remember all the time and deep breathing it took to unravel it? It is the same principle with carbs: the more complex the chain, the longer it takes to unravel, making complex carbs a much better choice than simple ones if you want sustained energy.

Examples of complex carbohydrates are:

- Quinoa
- Oats
- Brown rice
- Rye/pumpernickel bread
- Pulses
- Sweet potatoes
- Beets

Choosing complex over simple avoids the dreaded sugar crash, so the best and most logical way to get more energy into your body is to slowly feed it into your system over a period of hours rather than dumping it in all at once.

The bottom line on carbohydrates is that without them your body and brain just don't work as well. Period. You need those good little guys to give you the energy currency you need to exist – it's simple science. Avoiding them means a lifetime of lethargy and misery; choosing the right carbs in moderation will promote long-term health, energy and happiness. Can't get clearer than that.

- Carbohydrates are simple or complex; the more complex they are, the longer they take to break down, giving you sustained energy. It is more beneficial for your overall wellbeing to switch from simple carbs to complex carbs.

- Good carbohydrates are an essential energy source and are crucial for your wellbeing, brain function and overall energy levels.

- Switch shop-bought cereal to oatmeal with berries and nuts.

- Switch white rice to brown rice.

- Switch white bread to rye/pumpernickel bread.

- Switch alcohol to kombucha.

- Switch sweet fizzy drinks to fizzy water.

- Switch ketchup to olive oil and balsamic vinegar.

- Switch chips to sweet potato wedges.

ARTIFICIAL SWEETENERS

Sometimes we get confused between weight loss and health. Trust me, they are worlds apart and artificial sweeteners are a great example. Due to their 'weight loss' benefits we assume that they must be good for us – not quite. Probably the most well-known artificial sweeteners are aspartame and sucralose. What is less well-known are the long-term effects these chemicals can have on our bodies. Although both of these are approved for consumption and considered safe at governmental level, there have been enough studies to suggest that these chemical substitutes are not good for you, and certainly enough evidence to dissuade me from consuming them. Furthermore, one of the best reasons to steer clear of artificial sweeteners is that if a food manufacturer thought it was a good idea to remove the natural sweetness and replace it with a chemical, chances are you're better off without it entirely. And to top it all off, in an ironic twist, research has suggested that sweeteners can cause overeating in some consumers. When it comes to common sugars and alternatives, sweeteners are considered the least healthy. That is because the jury is out on these, so when in doubt, cut it out!

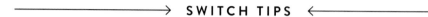

SWITCH TIPS

- Avoid sweeteners like sucralose and aspartame and switch to the most natural of sweeteners – stevia, which is derived from a plant.

- Switch white sugar or brown sugar to natural sweeteners such as agave syrup or coconut sugar.

WHAT THE HELL IS THE GI TABLE?

GI stands for glycaemic index. Put simply, it tells you how quickly a carbohydrate will process in the body. Remember, the slower a carbohydrate processes, the better it is for your body. The GI figure is calculated by watching the effect of the level of sugar on the body, and assigning it a number between 1 and 100. Stick to lower GI-numbered carbs for normal daily activities; however, if you are partaking in rigorous sports, consume foods with higher GI levels, as they will give you more energy. Just be careful to not overindulge with foods that are high on the glycaemic index if you are not being physical.

EXAMPLES OF LOW-GI FOODS:

- **BREADS** – dark versions such as wholegrain, multigrain, rye and sourdough
- **CEREALS** – porridge made with rolled oats, quinoa, barley or buckwheat
- **PASTA AND NOODLES** – wholewheat pasta, soba, vermicelli and rice noodles
- **FRUIT** – apples, dark berries, apricots, peaches, pears
- **VEGETABLES** – carrots, broccoli, cauliflower, celery, courgettes, sweet potatoes
- **PULSES** – lentils, chickpeas, butter beans, kidney beans
- **DAIRY** – cows' milk, soya milk

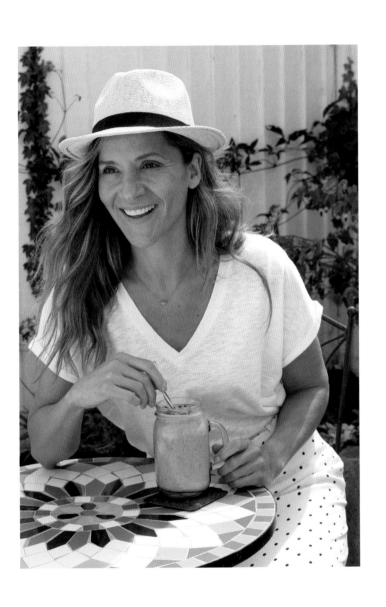

- **BREADS** – white bread, bagels, naan bread, French baguettes
- **CEREALS** – instant oats, any sugary cereals such as Cheerios
- **PASTA AND NOODLES** – white pasta and instant noodles
- **FRUIT** – watermelons, raisins
- **VEGETABLES** – boiled or mashed potatoes
- **SAVOURY SNACKS** – rice crackers, pretzels
- **CAKES AND BISCUITS** – scones, doughnuts, cupcakes, cookies, waffles
- **DAIRY** – rice milk

Remember, foods such as meat, fish, nuts, oils and herbs that contain few or no carbohydrates will not have a number on a GI list.

THE SKINNY ON FAT

—

Let me get one thing clear; *dietary fat* and *body fat* are two completely different things. And yet, we have been programmed into thinking that dietary fat should be avoided at all costs. While there is no doubt that there are bad dietary fats, there are many good dietary fats that are essential when it comes to the smooth function and metabolism of the body. The trick is to know your good from your bad.

UNSATURATED FATS

These come in two forms: monounsaturated and polyunsaturated. Unsaturated fats are found in:

- Nuts and seeds
- Vegetable oils
- Oily fish

ESSENTIAL FATTY ACIDS (EFAS) are called essential because our bodies cannot make them; hence it is 'essential' to get them from your diet. EFAs are found in:

- **FISH** such as tuna and salmon (only eat small amounts of tuna as it is high in mercury)
- **EGGS** (preferably organic)
- **NUTS AND SEEDS** such as cashews, almonds, Brazil nuts, pumpkin and sunflower seeds (not roasted, salted or flavoured)
- **AVOCADOS** contain oleic acid – a fatty acid that is linked to reduced inflammation and has been shown to have beneficial effects on genes linked to cancer
- **OILS** such as olive, flax seed, avocado and algal oil (a by-product of algae that is rich in omega-3 oils – a vegan source of omega-3 if you do not want to eat fish)
- **FLAX SEEDS**, **WALNUTS** and **CHIA SEEDS** are rich in omega-3 fatty acids – in fact, chia seeds contain more omega-3 than salmon, gram for gram

SATURATED FATS

While a balanced diet does include some saturated fats, an excess intake has been linked to health problems such as heart disease and some forms of cancer. Sat fats are found in:

- **MEAT** (fatty cuts of beef, pork, lamb)
- **PROCESSED MEATS** (salamis, sausages)
- **DAIRY** (butter, cream, milk, ghee, cheese)

TRANS FATS

These are the baddest boys of the fat world, mostly because they are mainly manufactured, and rarely occur naturally. The worst thing about trans fats is that they are made to extend the shelf life of products, so they are extremely processed and toxic. These little bastards are so bad for you and can cause such a range of health issues, there have been calls for them to be banned in the food industry altogether. So try to steer clear as often as you can from the following:

- Crisps
- Ready meals
- Fast food
- Chips
- Crackers
- Biscuits

- Cakes
- Frozen pies
- Pastries and muffins
- Margarine
- Snack foods, including microwave popcorn

→ **SWITCH TIPS** ←

- There are three types of fat: unsaturated (including EFA), saturated and trans fats.

- Saturated fats should be eaten in small amounts.

- Trans fats are the naughty fats and to be avoided at all costs.

- Healthy fats keep you fuller for longer. They take much longer to enter the bloodstream, which can in turn help you to get off the sugar rollercoaster that makes you crave a sweet snack a few hours after your meal.

- If taken in moderation, good fats can actually aid weight loss.

- Switch margarine or low-fat spreads to smaller amounts of full-fat butter.

- Switch butter on toast to avocado on toast.

- Switch roasted and salted nuts to raw, unsalted nuts.

PROCESSED FOODS

—

Processed foods are foods that have been processed to alter them from their original state. Natural, non-processed foods are nutritionally dense and will feed your body with oodles of nutrients that will help to keep you slim and healthy. However, in their altered or processed states, nutrients are lost, and they contain extra artificial ingredients, often making them counterproductive for our health.

We can feel frustrated if food goes off quickly, for example when that lovely artisan sourdough you bought two days ago turns rock hard or mouldy. But the fact is, if food goes stale or goes off quickly, you know it is good food. Food that stays fresh for a long period of time can only mean one thing: it is laced with preservatives, chemicals and additives to make it last longer, additives that are hazardous to our health.

Eating processed foods can cause inflammation and disease and a whole host of issues including anxiety, bad skin and, in some cases, even depression. So try to avoid them as much as possible.

$\longrightarrow$ SWITCH TIPS $\longleftarrow$

- Stick to foods that have been picked from a tree, have come straight from the ground, have been able to fly, swim, or graze the land and that are in as close to their original state as possible.

- The best food is fresh and probably doesn't have a label.

- Switch breaded chicken Kiev to grilled chicken breast.

- Switch vegetable tempura to steamed or roasted veggies.

- Switch sugary jam to mashed berries.

- Switch tinned tuna to tuna steak.

- Switch fish fingers to pan-fried cod fillet.

- Switch creamy coleslaw for grated salad.

WHAT IS FIBRE (AND WHY DO I NEED IT)?

—

Fibre comes from plants. It doesn't contain calories and cannot be digested by the human body – instead it passes through our digestive system and gives it a good clean on the way through, removing waste efficiently. Getting rid of toxic, potentially harmful waste is important so you want to give your body the best tools with which to maintain a healthy colon and prevent potential disease. Fibre comes in two forms: soluble and insoluble.

❶ SOLUBLE FIBRE DISSOLVES EASILY IN WATER. It can be found in oat bran, barley, nuts, seeds, beans, lentils, peas, and some fruits and vegetables. Psyllium husk is a good supplement to take if you feel you do not get enough fibre.

❷ INSOLUBLE FIBRE DOES NOT DISSOLVE IN WATER. It is found in foods such as wheat bran, vegetables and whole grains.

The reason they say that fibre keeps you 'fuller for longer' is because it takes the body longer to process it than other foods, plus it is bulkier and therefore stays in your stomach longer.

There are other cool things that fibre can do. It slows down the absorption of carbohydrates, which in turn reduces their effect on our blood sugar levels and maintains a healthy weight in return, and it can lower LDL (bad) cholesterol levels and also aid in ridding excess hormones, which can improve fertility levels – yeah baby!

The main sources of dietary fibre are fruits, vegetables and cereals, hence the well-known, worldwide five-a-day campaign.

- To make sure you are packing your diet with a fibrous punch, switch sugary cereals to wholegrain breakfast cereals, white pasta to wholewheat pasta, white bread to wholegrain bread, fruit juice to whole fruits and mash to jacket potatoes (skin included). When it comes to vegetables, the darker the vegetable, the higher the fibre content.

- Foods that are dense in fibre take the body longer to digest and help to keep you fuller for longer. They take much longer to enter the bloodstream, which can in turn help you get off the sugar rollercoaster that makes you crave sweet snacks a few hours after your meal.

- Increase fibre where possible. A regular orange or banana will take care of two portions, so having enough fibre in your diet should not be daunting or unattainable.

- While frozen fruit and vegetables are just as beneficial as fresh ones, the same cannot be said for dried fruits, processed fruit juices and yoghurt containing fruit.

LISTENING TO YOUR BODY'S LANGUAGE:

FOOD INTOLERANCES

—

Translating the language your body is speaking to you is an important part of understanding how it works.

Think of yourself as a translator at the UN summit. Your job is pretty important because what you interpret someone saying could mean the difference between World War III and world peace. In the same way, when you translate how your body feels after certain foods, it could mean the difference between feeling bloated, ill, having bad skin or gaining or losing weight (not quite WW III but you catch my drift). Eventually, your mind and body will realise that they can trust your instincts, and that healthy eating should be celebrated and not feared.

LACTOSE

Reactions to food intolerances are a good example of the language your body speaks to you. Let's take lactose – a sugar found in milk and other dairy products. There has been a lot of research done to prove that a high proportion of us do not digest lactose properly. The effects of this are that the immune system treats lactose (sugar molecules, to be precise) like space invaders. Space invaders come crashing into the body shooting their sugary molecules all over the place, leading to explosions in the system such as wind, bloating and even diarrhroea. Now this is pretty loud and expletive-filled body language, yet often we ignore it (erm, how loud does it have to shout or how stinky does the stink bomb have to be before you listen to it?) Until you experiment with eliminating something like lactose from your diet, you will never be able to associate your symptoms with the culprit.

FRUCTOSE

I discovered over time that I am intolerant to fructose (the natural sugar contained in fruit). I know this because when I eat dried or super-sweet fruits, like apples, mulberries, dried apricots or raisins, my husband is tempted to sleep in the spare room. The irony of how sweet these foods are in comparison to the nasty smell that they make me emit is not lost on me. I resisted for a long time the fact that I was potentially intolerant to these foods, but that was probably because I was single and it didn't matter how bloated or smelly I was. I mean, if a tree falls in the wood and there is no one there to hear it, does it really make a sound? But when you have a husband to consider, sleeping in the same bed beats that bowl of blueberries every time.

WHEAT AND GLUTEN

Other culprits you may want to consider are wheat and gluten, mostly found in bread and pasta. Symptoms of intolerance include bloating, pain, tiredness and even depression. So if you often feel bloated after a meal, and you haven't eaten *that* much, try to think about what you ate when you had that reaction. Was it pizza or a bowl of pasta? The bloating could be because of *what* you ate, not how much.

So tune into what you are being told by your body, by experimenting and cutting out all the unnecessary (foods that contain no nutritional value) or unhealthy parts of your diet. Start to eliminate, one by one, things that you think may be causing you to be intolerant, and then re-introduce them again, and you may be surprised at what you find, how you feel, and how fresh you smell!

OUR BODIES = GLORIOUS MACHINES

Food is so much more than just the fuel we put into our bodies; it contains a story. Every choice you make to eat something sets off a chain reaction in the body, meaning that we each have the ability to create healthy bodies just by the food choices we make – cool, huh? The chemical reactions that food triggers throughout the body include making hormones, cleaning the mess that dead cells leave behind (dirty buggers), switching gene cells off and on and managing our immune systems. Christ, our bodies are such well-structured wonders that I am surprised we don't stand in front of the mirror all day chanting 'All Hail, The Bodacious Body!' (Homework: do that tonight.)

The very notion that we beat ourselves up over these glorious machines, and the notion that we have such unhealthy relationships with the magical food we put into them is crazy. They deserve to be treated with the utmost respect. I hope you see now why it is important to understand the value of food and to love your body enough that you want it to be healthy and happy. Appreciating food for what it is, and taking away the fear surrounding it, is the key to a long-term happy relationship with food and your body.

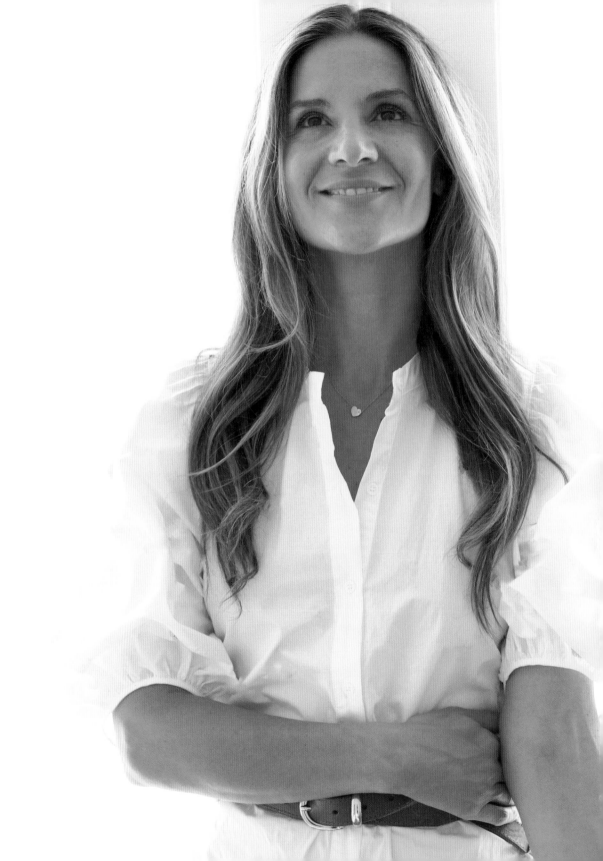

'CAN I JUST TAKE A
MOMENT TO REMIND
YOU: YOU ARE JUST
AS FUN, FUNNY AND
CONFIDENT WHEN YOU
ARE SOBER!'

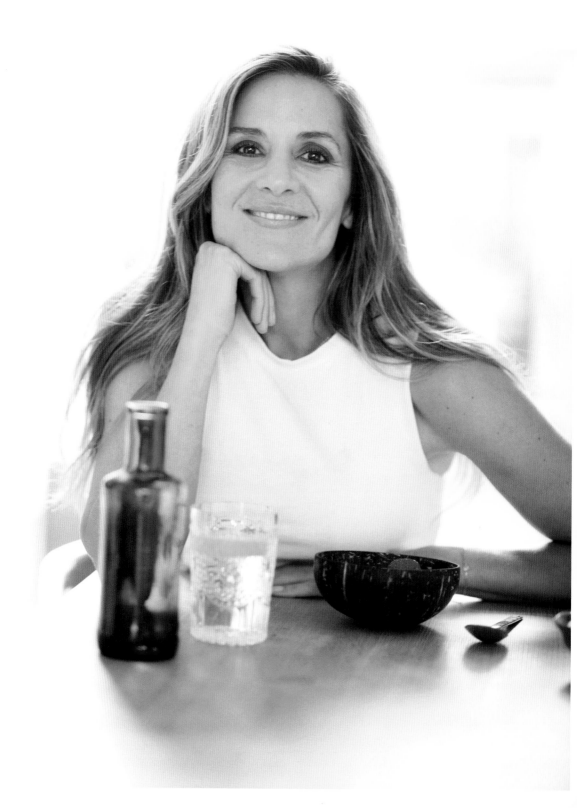

SADs:

SUGAR, ALCOHOL

AND DRUGS

⟵⟶

IN THE COURSE of our lives we come into contact with things that we will think will make us happy but ultimately can leave us feeling a little SAD. I am of course talking about sugar, alcohol and drugs or, as I call them, SADs. Just a note; when I say drugs I mean any mind-altering chemical, including caffeine. So in this section I'll examine ways in which SADs affect your body and offer a few suggestions on how to kick the habits for good.

THE EFFECTS OF SUGAR ON THE BODY

—

It is really important to understand how our bodies process sugar and by sugar, I don't mean complex carbohydrates, I mean the sweet, white, addictive powder most of us have in our cupboards. The most obvious side-effect of eating too much sugar is weight gain, but did you know the plethora of other bodily functions sugar can mess with? The truth isn't so sweet.

1. BRAIN FUNCTION

Sugar acts like a drug, fuelling our brain with a surge of dopamine, the same chemical that is released if you were to take that other white powder ... cocaine! And much like Columbian marching powder, in the absence of the drug, your brain will crave it fiercely. We have all heard that post dinner voice on our shoulder whispering sweet-Häagen-Dazs-nothings softly into our ear. Unfortunately sugar is so addictive that the more you eat, the stronger the cravings get.

2. SKIN CONDITION

There is no easy way to say this, except that sugar causes inflammation and ageing. It creates harmful molecules called 'advanced glycation end products' which (in plain English) means that it damages precious collagen and elastin, the two things we need to keep skin young and plump.

3. BUZZ KILL

Sugar gives you a high when it raises blood sugar levels. But what goes up must come down; and once that spike disappears, 'the crash' happens (enter Miss Grumpy Pants). Moreover, there have been multiple links observed between excess sugar intake and a risk of depression. Not so sweet at all.

4. PANCREAS AND DIABETES

The pancreas controls our blood sugar levels. If you overindulge on sugary things, it is likely that you will have trouble controlling your weight. Having excess weight is a strong risk factor for type 2 diabetes because the pancreas is no longer able to control blood sugar levels, leading to an increased risk of many other chronic health problems.

5. SWEET HEART

Excess sugar intake can affect the arteries in your heart meaning that, over time, the heart can become damaged, which can lead to heart disease, heart attacks or strokes.

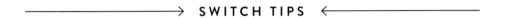

SWITCH TIPS

- Switch table sugar to natural alternatives such as xylitol or stevia.

- Switch sugar on your morning porridge to agave syrup or coconut sugar.

- When baking try to switch table sugar to more natural alternatives, such as agave syrup, coconut nectar or maple syrup, or use half sugar and half apple sauce.

- Be mindful of the *type* of sugar you are eating (see page 44).

- Be aware of *how much* sugar you are eating.

- Always keep in mind the effect sugar is having on your body, such as your brain, skin, energy levels, pancreas, liver and heart. That should help you to remember the reasons why too much is not good for you.

THE TRUTH ABOUT ALCOHOL

—

EXPLICIT WARNING: The following content may leave you with feelings of dread and fear – some of this knowledge could be life-changing.

DISCLAIMER: I was once a groaner. Now I am groan-free, fun, confident AND still drink the odd time.

THE GROAN SYNDROME*

Note: The Groan can also be substituted with an upward-to-heaven eye roll.

The Groan is that sound I just heard you make as you read the title of this chapter. Yes you. Trust me, I totally, totally, totally (there actually aren't enough 'totallys' to convey just how much) get it. I was the biggest groaner of all time. Booze was my bestie, my dancing partner, and my confidant. Most of all, it was my social crutch. I was the first girl to buy a round and I was the last girl standing (usually on a table or a chair) ordering shots for the group. I was a fan of drink and I was a fan of getting drunk. However, I wasn't a fan of the hangover that seemed to just get worse and worse as each birthday passed. And I certainly wasn't a fan of the inexplicable softness around my belly and the cellulite that seemed to get worse when I drank excessively. I finally realised that it was probably the vodka and wine playing havoc with my lumps and bumps; after all, alcohol is pure sugar.

On the other hand, the thought of cutting back on, or (God forbid) giving up alcohol filled me with absolute abject terror in a way I cannot explain. It was almost as terrifying as the fear of death. I mean if I am not drinking I might as well be dead, right? What is the point in being on this earth if you can't get utterly wasted and tell everyone how much you love them, even when you can't remember their name the next day? For so many of us, the thought of not drinking alcohol is so abhorrent that it immediately activates ... The Groan Syndrome.

So often women come to me and say, 'Help! I just can't lose weight no matter what I do. I would do anything, and I mean ANYTHING to lose weight.' To which I reply, 'Have you tried cutting out drinking for two weeks, or even cutting down drinking to Christmas, birthdays, weddings and funerals?' They often go quiet and regard me with puppy-dog eyes, silently pleading for a better answer. I'm sorry, gang, I hate to strut into the party, pull down my pants and piss in your Pinot Noir, but drinking even small amounts of alcohol on a regular or semi-regular basis really messes with your system.

When I eventually hear The Groan and get reminded (quite sharply) that 'life is too short to give up booze for even just one week!' my immediate reaction is: 'Some of you have pushed a 10lb screaming baby out of your vagina so I am pretty sure abstaining for a few days would be easy in comparison!'

SO WHY DO WE GROAN?

Truth is like poetry, and most people fucking hate poetry.
(THE BIG SHORT)

We all know that cutting back on booze is probably a great idea if we want to lose weight, stay in shape and stay healthy. Yet the announcement that someone in your friend group is not drinking, or when someone, or some article, informs us that booze is not good for our physique or for our general health, we want to punch someone in the tits. More often than not, said article gets brushed past quickly or thrown in the recycling bin, never to be read – because if you don't read it, it doesn't exist and therefore is not true. Right?

It is important to ask yourself the question, 'Why do I groan or roll my eyes when someone tells me I should quit or cut back on alcohol?' The answer is most likely to be the fear of not being allowed to have a 'social crutch' and the belief that alcohol makes us fun, funnier and confident.

Can I just take a moment to remind you: **YOU ARE JUST AS FUN, FUNNY AND CONFIDENT WHEN YOU ARE SOBER!**

Despite this truth, we believe wholeheartedly that booze is the 'personality juice' that enables us to make the first move, to say what we want to say to whoever we want to say it to (even if we regret it), and to make us feel relaxed and part of a social circle of fun people. We don't want to be the party pooper, the one who is left in the corner, the reject who didn't get picked for the PE team or the weirdo who is happy to have a laugh without being drunk. We want to bring the party, be part of the party, we actually want to BE the party. We want to be loved for our fun-ness and our ability to drink everyone else under the table.

We especially love it when people say they love the 'drunk us'. 'Drunk Amanda' was a firm favourite among pals, whether she was at a social event or a dinner party, drinking cider with friends in the summer sunshine or clinking a glass of champagne to celebrate something ... anything. It was especially hard in my industry, where 'showbiz' functions and events are obligatory. I realised that I would enter one of these intimidating rooms, immediately ask where the bar was, and then make a panicked beeline to it.

We've all been there, I mean God forbid we have to spend 10 minutes making idle chat with a stranger or even a 'friend', without a glass in our hand. If you had told me that alcohol was having a negative effect on my moods, or that it was probably why I was gaining weight around my abdomen, or adding to my cellulite – I WOULD HAVE GROANED loudly right in your stupid know-it-all face.

But I knew that alcohol was not the answer, hard as that was to admit. And I also knew that it was affecting my skin, my weight and my midweek mood. Plus, as I got older, the after-effects of a night out started to affect my whole week. So I quit. And guess what … I didn't die! (Thank God or that would have been mortifying: 'TV PRESENTER DROPS DEAD AFTER FIRST NIGHT OFF BOOZE'.)

I will admit I did find social occasions really hard and for the first few months I stayed away from big events. But slowly, I learned to love being in a room without a glass in my hand, because I became more confident that I was just the same person with or without a drink. Of course I lost friends along the way, who were my 'party pals'. They slowly stopped inviting me to occasions and dinner parties, which was hurtful at first but I realised that it was not about me; it was about them, because my abstinence was making them feel uncomfortable.

It was helpful that my husband and I had both decided to pull away from alcohol not long before we met, which made having sober dates in a brand-new relationship much easier – a unique experience. The fact that we didn't have that alcohol 'crutch' in the early days meant we formed a relationship that was based on plain old-fashioned sober conversation!

With all that said, I am not teetotal. I do have the odd drink, but these days it is extremely rare and I can do this because I learned how to be OK without alcohol. I don't feel a dark cloud of social fear hanging over my head any more. Over time I learned how to relax in a room with or without a drink, and so 99 per cent of the time now, I choose not to drink.

If we are with our friends, family and people we love, then why do we need alcohol to make us feel like we are more interesting people to be around? All too often, the opposite is true – when we are drunk, we forget sentences, we mix up stories, and we dismiss important conversations.

I am not going to spend time telling you not to drink, or that Mary gained a shitload of weight from all the boozing she was doing or Rachel lost a ton of weight by quitting booze for a month. Instead, I'm going to explain to you the science behind weight and alcohol and the physiological chain of events that happen to our bodies when we drink. Life would be long and void of fun if we were never allowed to drink ever again if we really wanted to, so it is important to be smart about the way you drink, how often you drink and what you drink.

WHAT IS ALCOHOL?

Alcohol is made as a result of the fermentation of sugars, therefore in plain English: alcohol is sugar. And since it is made of mainly sugar, it is highly calorific.

Forget liquid lunches and boozy diets to 'keep the calorie intake down'; alcohol contains 'empty calories', meaning there is ZERO nutritional benefit to be gained from drinking it – soz about that. As I explained in 'The effects of sugar on the body' (see page 49), this little white powder can have a devastating effect on our bodies. But the 'drink booze = gain weight' equation is not that black and white. There are many processes in place that lead to weight gain from alcohol, and they mostly have to do with your liver and your hormones. I won't get too scientific (even though the science bit is fascinating!), but it is important for you to know a few basics before making your own choices or alterations around alcohol.

HORMONE DISRUPTION AND WEIGHT GAIN

Let's start with the endocrine system. This brilliant and intricate system is a hormone regulator, kind of like a parent dishing out pocket money, making the kids happy, helping them to grow and making sure they get enough sleep, food, drink and fun. It allows the body to be able to cope with both internal and external mechanisms and is responsible for our mood, body growth, metabolic function, breakdown of important nutrients and sexual development. This system can only operate smoothly when there are clear lines of communication between the nervous system, the immune system and the body's circadian rhythms. However, when we drink alcohol these lines of communication can get fuzzy and disrupted, causing short- and long-term damage to our bodies.

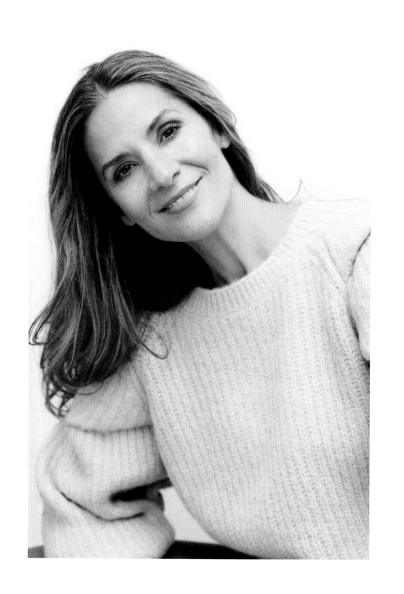

HORMONES: THE KEY PLAYERS

Alcohol can interfere with the adequate function of hormones, and the top dogs are: cortisol, vasopressin, insulin and oestrogen.

- **CORTISOL** – levels of this hormone that deals with stress increase when you drink alcohol. This not only happens when you are drinking, but also in the 'aftermath' – the hours and days afterwards. This has short- and long-term effects. Short term, it increases blood pressure and encourages belly fat because that is where cortisol likes to hang out. And long term, both digestive and reproductive systems can suffer.
- **VASOPRESSIN** – drinking alcohol reduces this antidiuretic hormone, which means the kidneys send water straight to the bladder instead of reabsorbing it into the body. That explains your non-stop visits to the little girls' room while on a bender, which leave you dehydrated the next morning.
- **INSULIN** – this is the hormone that is responsible for regulating your blood sugar levels. Because alcohol's sugar content is so high it sends your insulin production into overdrive, in turn messing with your blood sugar levels.
- **OESTROGEN** – normal levels of oestrogen are perfectly fine; it is the hormone that makes us 'women' in the 'women' department. But when we drink alcohol it is thrown out of sync and increased oestrogen can cause havoc in the 'Fat Department'.

PROCESSING THE POISON

Your liver is your powerhouse organ; when operating smoothly it is a fat-burning machine. It is where carbs get broken down and turned into the body's energy currency, glycogen. It is the also the Henry of vacuums, the Dettol of multipurpose cleaners and the car wash that brushes all the grime from your car after you've been on a messy drive through the muddy fields. This is because the liver is second to none at excreting hormones and toxins (everything from sugar to alcohol and drugs) and all the crap we put into our bodies. It is the body's own detox centre and its numerous functions are crucial to a healthily regulated body. Consuming alcohol can put a big spanner in the liver's works.

Picture the scene: you have had your first drink of the evening and, naturally, you opt for a gin and slimline tonic. After all, it's the healthy choice, right? Cut to the end of the night when, after several hours of slamming G&Ts, you're ready for some bad dietary choices: a kebab, a plate of cheesy chips and a large helping of that chocolate cake you've been craving all week. Normally, your blow-out feast would send your body into overdrive as it attempts to process all the calories in your high-carb and high-fat midnight meal. However, given that alcohol is also dense with calories, your body is now faced with a choice: either use the calories in the booze or the calories in the food. It's a no-brainer, because the booze is a poison which your body must detoxify in order to stay alive, so of course it opts to rid itself of the toxin, storing the cake and kebab to be dealt with another day.

FERTILITY ISSUES AND BREAST CANCER

Drinking too much can impair the function of the ovaries, resulting in hormone deficiencies and potential fertility issues. Some people can experience sexual dysfunction, and that is a REAL buzz kill.

Alcohol-induced raised oestrogen levels can create symptoms of polycystic ovary syndrome, endometriosis, fibroids and worse. Also studies have shown that increased oestrogen can cause breast cancer. A study done in the UK by the NHS showed that there is an increase of breast cancer among women who drank heavily in their youth.

ALCOHOL AND BLOOD SUGAR FUNCTION

The reason you will feel hungrier the more you drink is because the metabolism of booze can mess with blood sugar levels by sucking up your storage of glycogen (the body's energy source). Since glycogen is formed from sugary foods and carbohydrates, that is what we crave when we are drinking or hungover. Also, remember I mentioned vasopressin, the antidiuretic hormone? This is the cause of dehydration – meaning we also crave salty foods during or after a drinking session. Cue the chip butties!!

MOOD KILL

While alcohol is often used as a way of improving mood and getting your personality juices flowing, drinking can also lead to behavioural inconsistencies.

Alcohol has an effect on your levels of dopamine and gamma-aminobutyric acid (GABA), neurotransmitters that play an important role in behaviour. Alcohol consumption floods the brain's reward centre with dopamine, which gives you that feeling of being 'buzzed'. Dopamine also activates memory, meaning you are reminded of that buzzy feeling, hence the desire for *more* alcohol. Over time, however, alcohol can cause dopamine levels to decrease, leaving you feeling in a slump and craving even more alcohol. Do the phrases, *'Is it the weekend yet?/Is it wine o'clock yet?'* ring a bell?

Similarly, GABA has a relaxing effect on the body and alcohol mimics the effects. Over-consumption of booze over time can over-work the GABA pathways and desensitise them, which in turn will leave you craving alcohol to get that fix of feeling relaxed and sedate. So, as you can see, drinking can seriously mess with the effectiveness of these neurotransmitters and over time can lead to heightened anxiety, aggression and even depression.

THE HANGOVER

When you are hungover, you are experiencing the after-effects of intoxication. Your body is in turmoil and shock from the effects of alcohol. The poor thing is literally fighting to shake off the symptoms, and very often we are not fully focused or back to 'normal' again for many days after a drinking session. The problem with this is that as a society that centres on weekend drinking, very often our bodies have just recovered from the full effects of last weekend's alcohol by the time it gets to Friday, and we kick off drinking again. Essentially, we can be living in a constant haze, with a low hum of white noise that I call 'The Tinnitus of Life' in the background, never fully catching up on deep sleep, never really fully energised throughout the day, or never being able to function without relying on stimulants and SADs.

BUT I AM YOUNG – CAN'T I DRINK WHAT I WANT?

I am afraid not, girls. According to a study that was published in the *American Journal of Preventive Medicine*, those who drink heavily when they are in their prime, young years, have a higher risk of gaining weight and being overweight when they are older. The study found that 'regular heavy episodic drinking in young adulthood is associated with higher risk of gaining excess weight and transitioning to overweight/obesity'.

SHOULD I BE WORRIED?

Apart from the health and weight implications, there are other times when you should consider a move away from alcohol. When you start to notice yourself saying things such as 'I need a glass of wine to wind down,' or 'I want a glass of champagne because I need to celebrate,' or 'I won't be able to sleep unless I have this drink,' it's time to examine the triggers that urge you to consume alcohol and see if you can find alternatives.

BENEFITS OF NOT DRINKING

WEIGHT LOSS: For all the reasons explained previously, not drinking without a doubt leads to a shift in body weight and body shape. Also, with all the hangover-free mornings, you will be less likely to make bad food choices and more motivated to get out and get active – headache-free!

NO HANGOVERS: I cannot begin to tell you the joy of this feeling. When you wake up with a clear head, you feel a sense of relief and achievement. It sounds crazy, but whether we like it or not, having a sober night is something to be applauded.

CLEAR SKIN: The effect of anything toxic in your system will always eventually affect your skin. So eliminating booze for a while or at least cutting back will reveal some significant changes in your appearance and it can take years off your face.

A CLEAR HEAD: Not drinking allows you to really focus on having a clear head. But be aware – sometimes this will bring up feelings of anxiety and past issues. Remember, it is common practice to drink to eliminate these feelings in the first place. When you are taking a break from the booze, it is a good idea to take long walks, meditate and exercise to help with any surge in negative emotions that you would usually have numbed with alcohol.

EYE CONTACT: When I gave up alcohol and was out socialising, I realised that I was having conversations that were not simply drunken and meaningless. I also found that I was making eye contact with people more often, which I had felt uncomfortable doing (or next to near impossible!) when I was drunk.

ACTIVE LIFE: You will find that you have much more energy when you don't drink and you will be eager (or at least more enthused) to get out and work out.

SOUND SLEEP: Alcohol disrupts sleep patterns, and in turn your circadian rhythms can be put out of whack. You will notice that the less you drink, the more deeply you will sleep and the more rested and energetic you will feel the next day.

BENEFITS OF DRINKING

I'm sorry to be the bearer of bad news, but the benefits of drinking alcohol are few and far between. Yes, red wine *does* contain antioxidants in resveratrol (the dark pigment in red grapes), but the levels are so slim that you would be better off eating a bunch of grapes to get the right dose of this disease-fighting antioxidant. If excess weight from drinking is your primary concern, then cut back and drink smartly. However, if you have other health concerns, be extra cautious before opening that bottle of booze.

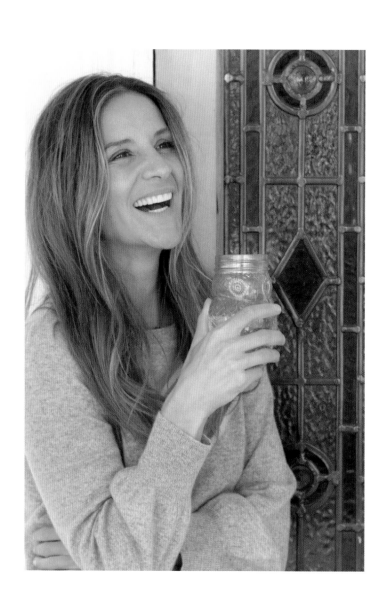

SWITCHING THE MINDSET ON ALCOHOL

—

If you really are serious about your health and your body and you are considering cutting back on alcohol for a few weeks, then you may find the following tips helpful:

- **NEVER SAY 'NEVER'** – telling yourself you can never drink again is a bad idea. You CAN drink if you want to, so if you really want something, denying yourself mentally will only make you want it more and indulge in unhealthy binge behaviour. The chances are, the less often you drink the less you will miss it.

- Give yourself **A TIMEFRAME** to begin with. Try quitting booze for 21 days. It has been proven that three weeks is the right timeframe to break addictive patterns.

- There will often be a **FRIEND DILEMMA** associated with cutting down or giving up alcohol – certain party-loving friends may be difficult to convince that this is the right thing for you. Whether they are jealous of your decision or they feel that you are a buzz kill, these types of friends will sabotage your efforts and try to shove a glass of vodka down your neck. These are the friends you should try to avoid at all costs during times of abstinence. You may want to retrospectively examine your circle of friends if they constantly mock you for not participating.

- If you are a part of a group that has drinking as a default activity every time you go out, why not start suggesting **ALTERNATIVE NIGHTS OF NON-DRINKING ACTIVITIES**? There are so many fun things to do that don't involve alcohol, and if these people are your friends, you should enjoy each other's company sober. Try booking an evening at the theatre, or go paintballing. Try a cookery course or rent a cottage by the ocean and take long walks. You never know, you may find that some of your pals want to join in, and were just waiting for the perfect excuse not to drink. You may be the catalyst that changes the dynamics of your friends' nights out – for the better.

- This one may seem a bit sneaky; however, in certain circumstances you may feel compelled to **JUST ORDER A DRINK** rather than announce, 'I am not drinking tonight.' Why create the (sober) elephant in the room? Simply order a drink and a glass of water too. Then sip the water in between times you are pretending to sip the alcohol. The drunker your friends get, the less they will care about whether you drink or not because they are now relaxed and don't really care about your drinking choices anymore. Soon you may notice your pals seem to be speaking in tongues – and there is a chance you will even seek out new friends after this experience, so be prepared to lose touch with certain buddies.

- If drinking is a stress reliever, **TRY TO REPLACE IT** with something that will *really* relieve stress, long-term. Try a walk in nature or five minutes of long, deep breathing (see chapter on Zen, page 165).

- If it is the 'ceremony' of opening the bottle that you enjoy, then when you finish a bottle of wine, **FILL IT WITH SPARKLING WATER** or a flavoured non-alcoholic drink and put it in the fridge. The next evening set the tone as usual – lighting a candle, playing your music to get 'in the mood' and pour the fizzy water, imagining it is wine. Examine if there is any part of you that is craving the 'ceremony' as opposed to the alcohol.

$$\longrightarrow \quad \text{S W I T C H   T I P S} \quad \longleftarrow$$

- For each alcoholic drink, have a glass of water.

- Dilute white wine with sparkling water.

- Switch tonic to sparkling water in your V&T and add a big squeeze of lemon juice. Lemons help to alkalise the body so this will help to balance the acidic environment in your body caused by the alcohol.

- Alcohol itself is calorific, so additives and mixers are a double whammy. Switch sugary mixers like Coke and fruit juices to sparkling water or sugar-free alternatives.

- Avoid cocktails completely – they are a sugar bomb nightmare.

- If you crack open the Rioja, only have one glass. Using alcohol as a stress reliever every time can be a slippery slope. Remember, it is a bottle full of sugar!

- If you do go out drinking, try to get to sleep on time and drink a pint of water before you do. If you know you will be home late, prepare your bedside table with a litre of water and make sure you drink it either before you shut your eyes or as soon as you wake up.

- Eat a good meal before you have your first drink. Alcohol hits the bloodstream with speed (that's the reason why some medicines are in an alcohol base).

And last, if you are contemplating giving up alcohol and are finding it hard to quit, ask yourself these two questions:

1. What does alcohol do for you: does it make you strong and clear, or does it make you weak and fuzzy?
2. Who has the power? If not you, do you really want alcohol to have power and control over you?

THE GREAT CAFFEINE DEBATE

—

Ah, caffeine ... that big daily cup of life-sustaining liquid that is responsible for an almost supernatural ability to run a marathon, catch up with your friends on email and write half a novel simultaneously. But why, then, is the recommendation to limit the amount we drink when studies have shown that caffeine is good for mental health and, in some cases, can possibly stave off Alzheimer's disease?

Let me start by saying, it is not caffeine *itself* that is bad for us; it is the *amount* of caffeine that we tend to drink. In the same way that a glass of wine may have slight antioxidant benefits, but a whole bottle will put your system out of whack (see page 57), excess caffeine can mess up your hormonal pathways, leading to feelings of irritability, disturbed sleep patterns and sometimes elevated heart rhythms.

If you are a caffeine lover, do you ever lie in bed at night wide awake, your heart racing, thinking to yourself, 'I shouldn't have had that third cup of coffee'? While you are no doubt aware that too much of your daily brew can cause a sleepless night, you might not know that things are also happening on a cellular level that can have long-term ramifications for your vitality, clarity and overall sanity!

Obviously, caffeine is a stimulant – it artificially increases your body's metabolism, so your body will have to deal with the consequences as well as working overtime to return to its natural and preferred state.

So what is actually going on inside when that morning Joe starts flowing through your veins? First, we need to consider the three hormones that are directly affected by that caffeine hit:

1. Adrenaline
2. Cortisol
3. Insulin

The rest is best explained with a story.

You are all dressed up in your summer frock and your new Aldo espadrilles. You look around and notice that everyone has disappeared, and in the distance you hear a faint scream ... suddenly, you realise that across the road just outside Zara there is a fully grown Bengal tiger on the loose and heading your way! Your body's immediate reaction is to FUCKING RUN and so you take off faster than Usain on his best day! As you sprint away (espadrilles now in hand), your adrenal glands go into overdrive and floods your system with the hormone adrenaline. This flooding is known as your 'fight or flight' response and within seconds, you'll be pumped up and ready for anything.

You sprint down the high street and take refuge in the first shop you can find. By the time you find yourself in the nightgown section in M&S, you realise you have shaken the aforementioned tiger and you are safe. Thank the Lord!

Now, as you are standing there considering why the hell there was a tiger on the high street (everyone knows that tigers shop online these days), your body has also been releasing a stress hormone called cortisol.

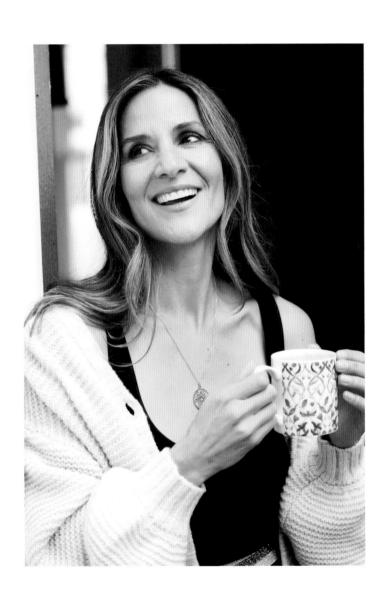

Cortisol primes your body to be more alert by increasing blood sugar levels and helping your body to use sugar more effectively, so that if the tiger reappears, you'll have enough energy to get away again.

With increased blood sugar, your body now pumps out insulin as a way of getting your levels back to a normal range, or possibly even lower than they were before before the tiger turned up and flashed his teeth. And this, my caffeine-loving chums, is what is commonly referred to as 'The Crash'.

Now replace the tiger with a cappuccino – the effect on your body will be similar if you over-consume caffeine. The artificial stimulation of your adrenal glands causes the same shock to your system because your body reads caffeine almost the same way as seeing the tiger, albeit a slightly less urgent rush. The hormones play the same role: the surge in energy is followed by the crash, and so we do what we think is best, which is either seek out sugary foods or head to the nearest coffee shop and get another cappuccino. Now, if you like your caffeine drink with all the trimmings, not only are you getting the blood sugar spike from the cortisol conversion, you are also getting a fast hit of sugar from the drink, resulting in even more strain on your system. And if all of that wasn't enough, cortisol has receptors in the abdomen, meaning an excess consumption of caffeine could lead to some unwanted and unexplainable belly flab.

If you find yourself in a cycle where you are having coffee to wake you up, crashing and then having more caffeine to wake you up again later in the day, then over time you could start to see some classic symptoms of adrenal fatigue:

- Difficulty waking up in the morning
- Extreme exhaustion
- Digestive issues
- Inability to handle stress
- A weaker immune system
- Constant cravings for caffeinated drinks to rectify the tiredness

In order to avoid the caffeine pitfalls, it is important to curb your enthusiasm for too many cups of coffee or tea. Switch a builder's brew to a green tea, a double espresso to a single or your midday cup of Joe to a matcha latte. While tea does contain caffeine, it has approximately half the amount that coffee has. Plus, green tea and matcha contain a healthy tannin called catechin – an antioxidant that is believed to reduce the risk of cancer. Last, don't have caffeine too late in the day: it will stop you getting a good night's sleep and the next day you'll be so tired that the only thing that wakes you up will be – yes, you've guessed it – more caffeine!

$\longrightarrow$ SWITCH TIPS $\longleftarrow$

- Try to stick to one cup of caffeine a day and switch any extra cups to other hot drinks instead, such as green tea. Although there is still caffeine in green tea, it also has high levels of antioxidants and that outweighs the fact that there is caffeine in it.

- Make an event of your one a day: mix up coffee shops, drink it slowly and enjoy every sip.

- Avoid the highly calorific creamy concoctions at your local coffee shop. It's better to add a little bit of full-fat cream, nut milk or even blend some unsalted butter with your coffee. A small amount of fat slows down the rate at which caffeine hits your system.

- If you are going to drink caffeine, try drinking it just before you work out – it will help you to get the best out of your session.

- Caffeine is a diuretic, meaning the more you drink the more you wee, so if you are going to drink coffee, make sure you stay hydrated.

- Stay as far away from energy drinks as you would the rogue tiger, because they are a disastrous concoction of caffeine and sugar that puts your body through hell.

- Stay away from diet pills – they are basically just concentrated caffeine (along with other stimulants). Their aim is to curb your appetite so you don't feel hungry, but as we have seen, the long-lasting side-effects of excess caffeine far outweigh the short-term fix.

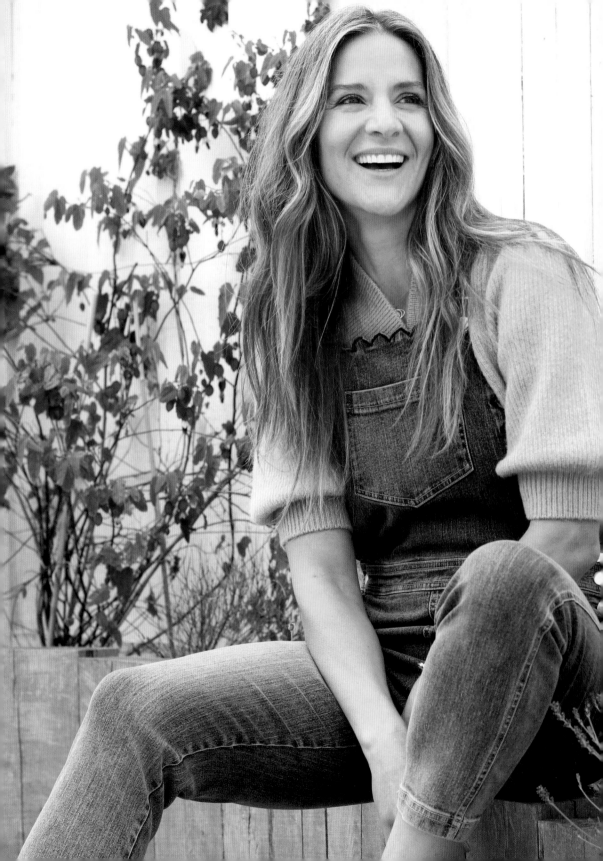

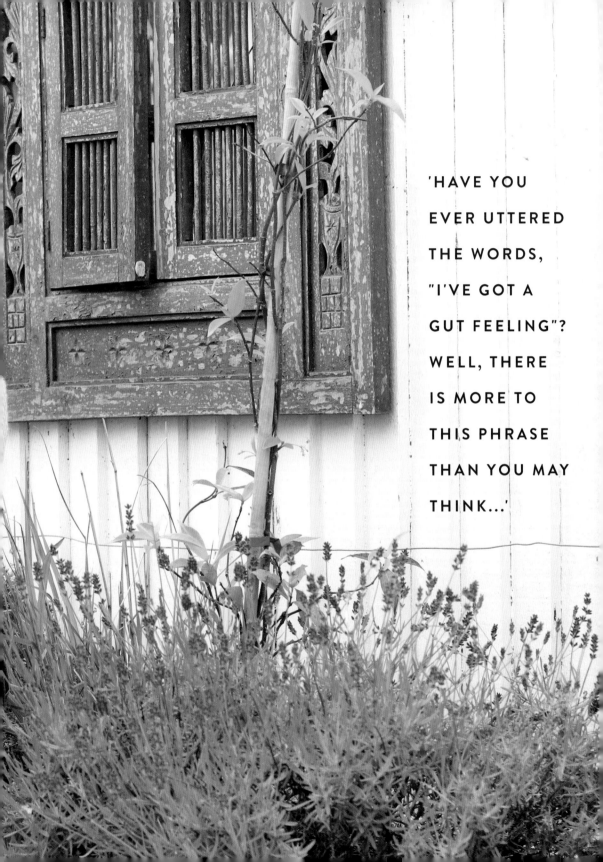

'HAVE YOU EVER UTTERED THE WORDS, "I'VE GOT A GUT FEELING"? WELL, THERE IS MORE TO THIS PHRASE THAN YOU MAY THINK...'

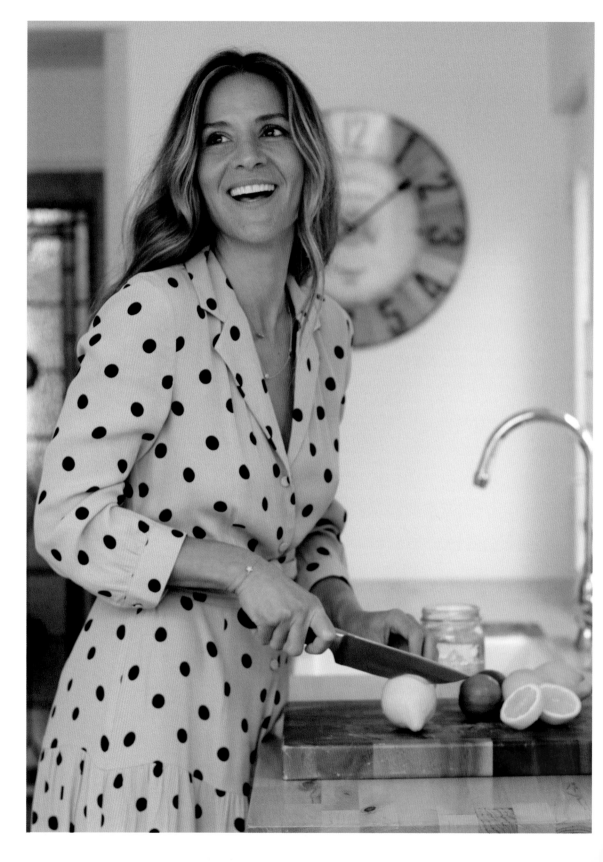

GUT

HEALTH

$\longleftrightarrow$

BY THE TIME YOU ARE BORN, you are already home to a unique ecosystem of trillions of single-celled organisms, collectively known as your microbiome. This complex profile of bacteria will stay with you for the rest of your life and this is where it gets crazy: for every human cell in your body, there are approximately three bacteria cells. To be more precise, human cells make up 43 per cent of the body's total cell count and the rest are microscopic colonists ... you do the maths ...!

Wait, I just did the maths and ... sweet holy Moses ... we are 57 per cent bacteria! MEANING WE ARE MORE MICROBIAL THAN WE ARE HUMAN! Now, ladies and germs, before you faint trying to calculate what that means for your sense of identity, let's swiftly move on to how this ecosystem works and what on Earth this could possibly mean for your health and wellbeing.

Well, like any complex society, the microbes that live inside us cluster and connect together to form neighbourhoods, towns and cities that co-exist in a delicate balance of daily life. As with every community, there are always a few rotten apples that cause havoc, but most of the bacteria that live in us are actually upstanding citizens, responsible for keeping us alive ... thanks, guys!

The capital city of this society of single-celled superheroes is without a doubt the human gut, and currently, within your digestive tract there are literally trillions of microbes congregating and doing everything from fighting disease to producing vitamins that affect your mood. That's right, they affect your mood and more than ever, we are waking up to the idea that our brains and these bacteria are linked in ways we cannot currently understand.

For instance, have you ever uttered the words, 'I've got a gut feeling'? Well, there is more to this phrase than you may think. Believe it or not, a network of neurotransmitters was discovered in the gut that acts in a similar way to ordinary neurons (like the ones in your noggin). This phenomenon is called 'the second brain', a term coined by American scientist Dr Michael Gershon in 1996. This network controls gut behaviour, dealing with gut issues independently of our brain. And get this: the brain in our heads is often informed about the rest of the body by our gut brain – isn't that mind-blowing? I am so proud of my little gut, standing on her own two (or trillions of) feet and making all these decisions for herself!

Even if you think this is far-fetched, the fact is that if you do not work in harmony with these little cities in your body, you could quickly wind up with rioting and civil unrest within. Indeed, an array of health complications including everything from inflammatory bowel disease to allergies to immune disorders and more are now being linked to gut health, not to mention high cholesterol, high blood sugar, mood swings, skin conditions and unexplained weight gain to boot.

In 2016 a scientific experiment was carried out by the US medical research agency the National Institute of Health. In the experiment, poo from lean or obese humans was transplanted into microbe-free mice, and lo and behold, the mice got thinner or fatter depending on whose microbiome they got! Now I understand that you might not fancy popping to your nearest hospital for a faecal implant (although I shit you not – pardon the pun – faecal micro-biota transplantations are becoming increasingly popular), so the best way to keep your gut bacteria in check is via your diet. As the Big Daddy of medicine Hippocrates once said, 'Let food be thy medicine and medicine be thy food.'

For ultimate gut health, there are three main components to focus on in the diet.

❶ First, your diet should be rich in **PREBIOTICS** to nourish existing good bacteria in the form of dietary fibre. These include a range of vegetables, berries, fruits, wholegrains and pulses (such as lentils).
❷ Then, to further boost your bacteria and keep your colony in good shape, take

daily **PROBIOTICS**. These are live bacteria found in fermented foods such as kefir, kombucha and sauerkraut. There are also many probiotic supplements available on the market nowadays.

❸ In addition, your gut bacteria love **POLYPHENOLS**, which are antioxidant-rich chemicals found in cloves, cacao, cherries, blackcurrants, blackberries, strawberries, raspberries, prunes and black grapes.

On the other hand, imbalances most commonly occur from over-use of antibiotics, which although a vital tool in the war against the bad guys, can also wipe out large populations of good bacteria. Think of it like dropping an atom bomb to catch a neighbourhood gang of ne'er-do-wells – sure, you caught the crims but at what cost? If you have recently taken antibiotics, you could remedy the situation by seeking out a good daily probiotic supplement that contains live activated cultures such as: *Lactobacillus rhamnosus, Enterococcus faecium, L. acidophilus* and *L. plantarum*.

Not only do antibiotics cause imbalances, there is an increasing body of evidence that in the western world, we are living on a daily diet that is working against our gut flora and undoing millions of years of evolution. Our ancestors enjoyed a microbiome that was diverse and robust because of their natural diet of 'living' foods instead of the tide of sweeteners, processed meals, chemicals and preservatives that now flood our food shelves and endanger our ancient internal residents. Ideally your daily diet should be like a cross between Gay Pride and the Chelsea Flower Show: colourful, alive and extremely diverse.

$\longrightarrow$ **SWITCH TIPS** $\longleftarrow$

- Don't be afraid of bacteria! Colonies of good bacteria are vital for your good health and are welcome microbes to have living inside you. In order to promote good gut bacteria, stock up on probiotics and prebiotics.

- Just as compromised gut health can affect your mood, a stressed-out mood can in turn affect your gut health – it's a two-way system. Try not to sweat the small stuff; try some of my tips for staying calm (see chapter on Zen, page 165).

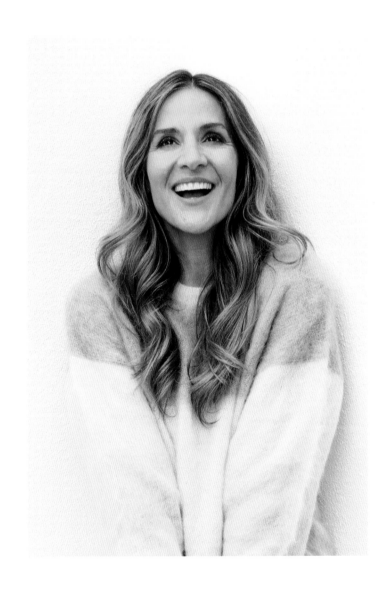

- Unless your doctor tells you that you absolutely *must* take antibiotics, steer clear of them, because they 'depress' your gut (cue bacteria slumped on a couch eating a tub of ice cream watching *Under the Tuscan Sun* for the trillionth time).

- The increasing use of chemical sanitisers not only wipes out the bad bacteria, it destroys the good bacteria too. Children's immune systems need to be 'trained' and the fewer microbes they are exposed to, the less 'training' their immune systems get. While the need to be clean and safe seems more important than ever since COVID-19, be mindful that excessive use could actually be affecting your child's immune system.

- Bacteria love fibre, so include plenty of wholegrains and pulses in your diet.

- Switch from sugary foods, processed foods, artificial sweeteners and unhealthy fats to plenty of fresh fruit and veg and fermented foods.

- Eat plenty of nuts and seeds – these also contain fibre, which help healthy gut bacteria to grow.

- Eat a diet rich in foods such as fresh lean meat, fish and good fats (like olive oil and avocado).

- Eat foods that are high in omega-3 (such as salmon or avocado). These foods have also been proven to be microbe- and brain-health-friendly.

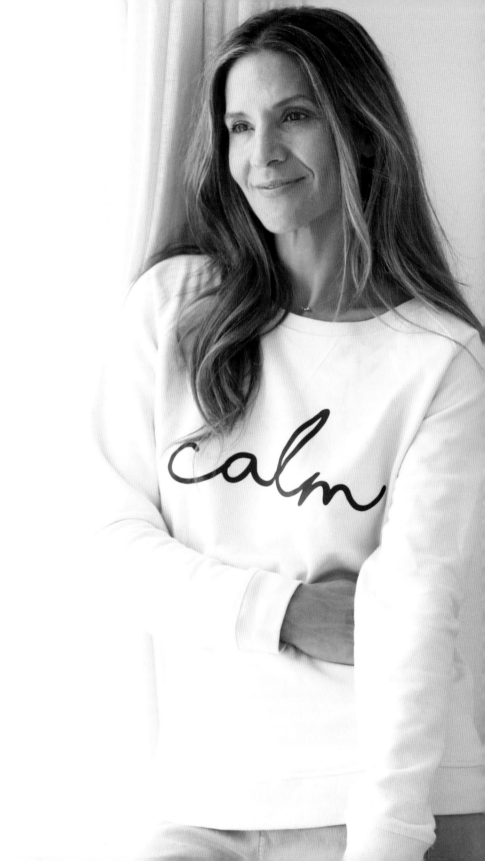

'CALL IT WHAT YOU WILL: INNER VOICE, MENTAL INTERCOM OR INNER CRITIC, VERY QUICKLY THE MENTAL CHATTER WE ALL EXPERIENCE REPLACES THE INNER QUIET AS AN ARRAY OF INTERNAL VOICES BEGIN TO PIPE UP AND COMMENT ON LITERALLY EVERYTHING WE THINK AND FEEL.'

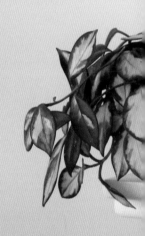

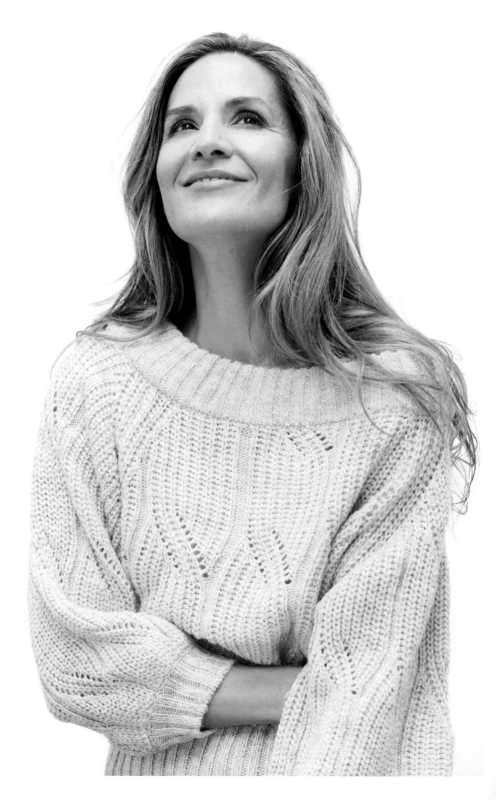

SWITCHING

THE

NARRATIVE

$$\longleftrightarrow$$

FEAR, GUILT AND SHAME

—

NOW WE'VE LEARNED about food groups and their physiological effects on the body, it's time to take that knowledge and put it into action. And in order to ensure that these thoughts can truly crystallise into long-lasting behavioural changes, it is imperative that we recognise the narrative we tell ourselves about eating and switch the emotions we experience with every meal, every morsel, and every moment we spend in the kitchen and beyond.

There is an innate sense of panic, fear, guilt and shame surrounding food and our bodies. I don't know where it all began, but I would like to revisit that moment in time and erase it. Since I do not own a DeLorean or a flux capacitor, I cannot do that, so the only way to eliminate the demons that exist in our heads is to understand what's going on with them, and why.

As soon as you clear the fog of panic, fear, guilt and shame about food and exercise from your head, you will find that you have more mental capacity to get that noggin of yours straight and realise that it is the 'fear' of being fat and out of shape that's crippling you.

If you fear weight and fear gaining it, then weight will hold on to you. If food and your body type are making you feel guilty, then it is not the food itself that is the problem; it is the feeling of guilt surrounding the food.

And if eating or not exercising is making you feel shame, it is not the eating or the lack of exercise that is crippling you; it is the feeling of shame.

In all three cases, it is neither you nor your weight that are the problem; it is the fear, the guilt and the shame of the weight.

Imagine there's a salted caramel choc chip cupcake on a plate in front of you. What goes through your mind? I am going to take a guess and say it is one of five things:

❶ Oh wow, that looks divine, I'm going to have that, but I need to eat it really quickly so that no one (including me) will see me eat it and therefore they cannot judge me for eating it.

❷ Oh wow, that looks divine, I could not possibly put that in my body, it's too fattening, it will dirty my insides plus I would never be able to wear my skinny jeans again.

❸ Oh wow, that looks divine, but I will have to work out extra hard this evening and for the rest of the week to get rid of the calories.

❹ I know I shouldn't do this, I am not sure why, but I can't help myself ... God help me.

❺ Oh wow, that looks divine, I cannot wait to treat myself to that when I fancy it, and after I have enjoyed every bite, I will go on and enjoy my day without giving it a second thought.

I imagine that 90 per cent of you went with thoughts 1 to 4? And those of you who chose one of the first four options will most likely have a habit of feeling fear, guilt or shame about food and body image. None of these emotions is healthy, and none of them will make you happy or enable you to be at peace with yourself or get to a place where you are in love with yourself, your food and your body.

Feelings of guilt around food are highly counter-productive. If you feel 'guilty' for having eaten something 'naughty', then your stress levels will rise. Guilt sounds a little bit like this:

'Crap, I really should not have eaten that salted caramel choc chip cupcake.'

Equally, shame is just as destructive – it runs deep, and is surrounded by feelings you have about yourself. Shame sounds a little bit like this:

'I am so bad for eating that salted caramel choc chip cupcake, I am a fat, stupid will-power-less moron.'

It is time for you to start being kinder to yourself and to your body. It's time to start letting go of the negative feelings. Fear, guilt and shame are emotions and feelings that we impose upon ourselves, meaning we can just as easily remove these feelings. Can you really have a little bit of everything and still maintain the shape you want? Well, yes mama, you can!

A well-balanced diet is part of a well-balanced lifestyle that will ensure that you can indulge in more pleasurable and less virtuous meals every now and then GUILT-FREE! As long as you have a balanced diet and you are not depriving yourself of the good stuff along the way, your body will settle down and understand what you are trying to do. Remember – do not stress about food, do not fear food, do not turn food into the enemy.

Overall, it is important to go easy on yourself, just as you would a child learning a new skill: take it slowly and make small changes at first. It is also important not to beat yourself up if you fall off the wagon and have a pizza slathered in chocolate spread. Just start fresh the following day and try harder.

The simplest path to unburdening yourself of these negative emotions is to re-train the way you think about food and the way you talk about food, both when speaking to yourself and others.

NEURO-LINGUISTIC PROGRAMMING

—

How we speak to ourselves makes all the difference to our mental health. There are so many ways we can switch the patterns of our internal voice to be more positive and productive, leading to a healthier happier you. The most famous is a technique called Neuro-Linguistic Programming (NLP) created by Richard Bandler and John Grinder in the 1970s. Simply put, NLP is the practice of programming the brain's language towards more strategic vocabulary for a more positive outcome.

'Neuro' refers to the brain and mind; 'linguistic' refers to language. The relationship between the two affects our behaviour, i.e. the 'programming'.

The mental strategies learned in NLP set those who practise it apart from the rest, helping them to learn faster and reach their fullest potential more quickly. You may have heard of some of the following NLP fans ... Oprah Winfrey, Bill Clinton, Tony Robbins, Russell Brand, Bill Gates, Tiger Woods and Robbie Williams.

Now ask yourself this: what do all of these people have in common? The answer is, 'success in their chosen field'. So you see, the way in which you speak to yourself, and also how you assimilate external influences into your own head, really makes a huge difference to your own behaviour.

Here are some tricks to talk yourself out of it when you hit a negative wall.

❶ You want to go to the gym, but you feel a little out of shape.

THE OLD NARRATIVE: 'I am fat, what's the point in going – I will look like a whale among all those beautiful women and everyone will laugh ... I might as well sit and watch daytime TV and eat those Cheesy Wotsits that have been screaming at me all week.'

THE NEW NARRATIVE: 'OK, you hot ball of sexy stuff, let's get this peachy butt to the gym, because you deserve to sweat, have fun, and kick some ass. Let's go, Lara Croft in the making!'

By eliminating any negative words or language here, you are simply not allowing yourself to believe the words and lies you berate yourself with. This means that the positive way in which you speak to yourself becomes a natural habit, and soon you'll be off to the shops to buy your Lara Croft get-up.

❷   Another common language mistake is telling or reminding ourselves how stressed we are:

THE OLD NARRATIVE: 'I am SO stressed out right now, my brain is so frazzled, I can't see straight. Has anyone ever died from stress? I think I am dying from stress.'

THE NEW NARRATIVE: 'I feel a little funky right now, so I am going to take a breath and see what happens.'

In the new narrative, changing the trigger word 'stress' to something a little more light-hearted makes all the difference. The more you tell yourself you are stressed, the more stressed you will become! You will find in time that by switching out negative words like stress, you will reprogram your mind into new ways of processing the world around you. Flip to the chapter on Zen to read more about stress management (see page 165).

❸   I often hear people repeat that they are filled with 'self-loathing'. By saying the words out loud you are reminding yourself that you loathe yourself, and this becomes a reinforcement that you do not like who you are.

THE OLD NARRATIVE: 'Ugh, I hate myself so much – my body, my hair, my mind. I am such a self-loather, that's just who I am, and it's not going to change.'

THE NEW NARRATIVE: 'The old me used to be so hard on herself, and that's not going to fly any more. I am bored of that narrative, it does not serve me, so you know what? I am one fucking foxy, funny, fabulous, fit, fantastic, fortuitous female ...'

THE VOICES IN OUR HEADS:

THE SOCK PUPPET

—

Right now, in your mind, you'll be listening to a voice as it reads the words appearing on this page. Of course, if you stop reading or the words simply run out, you'll be greeted by silence ... but not for long.

Call it what you will: inner voice, mental intercom or inner critic, very quickly the mental chatter we all experience replaces the inner quiet as an array of internal voices begin to pipe up and comment on literally everything you think and feel. Now while you have known these voices your whole life, that doesn't necessarily make them life-long friends – in fact, a few of these voices will treat you with such disdain, disrespect and degradation that you might be ashamed to utter some of the things they say to you. These negative voices know your innermost secrets and therefore what buttons to push in order to trigger a response. They know what decisions you'll make and can even create situations in your mind that do not exist in the real world.

They'll say things such as:

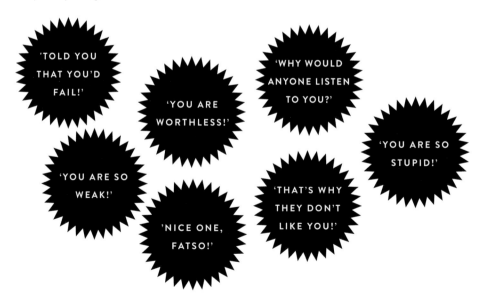

The list is endless and if left unchecked, this tornado of mental chatter can be all-consuming and take over our lives by sabotaging our outlook, depressing our mood, elevating anxiety levels and lowering self-esteem.

The most frightening part is that as we get older, our personalities change depending on which voices we listen to the most, and in some cases the voices can get so loud that we no longer hear what is happening in the outside world and disregard anything that might contradict or disprove what these voices are telling us.

If this sounds like it might describe your current state, then please know that it doesn't have to stay like this. As children, most of us were showered with praise and these positive outside voices always won over any inner doubts. Subsequently, we believed we were the best because pretty much every adult who cooed and clapped our every move reinforced this message day in, day out. Wasn't it nice to know that we pooed the best, came down that slide better than any other kid in the playground and were the best at finishing our vegetables at dinner? Wasn't it great when we sang that slightly tuneless song for our doting aunties and uncles and we were treated like four-year-old prodigies?

But fast-forward a few decades, and the unconditional approval many of us experienced as kids has long since evaporated. Instead our minds are awash with every conflict, cross word, rejection and remark that has ever been hurled in our general direction. We have forgotten the state of blissful positivity we used to thrive on. Worse still, our inner voices now have ample ammunition with which to fire bitchy bullets at us. Thankfully, this state does not have to be permanent and there is a simple fix to help rid ourselves of those negative demons once and for all.

First, acknowledge the negative voices and give them a singular identity. I imagined that my nasty, grouchy, hurtful voices were all wrapped up in a puppet from a kids' TV show. Introducing 'Mrs Zippy'...

When I was kid I used to watch the British TV show *Rainbow*. There was a glove puppet on it, Zippy, who had a zip instead of a mouth. Zippy would never shut up and was always being a bit of a nasty, cynical and controlling arsehole to Bungle the hippo and George the bear. Well, my puppet was the same, just a bitchy, mean-girl version ... and she was in my head, all the time.

For all intents and purposes, it was me controlling the puppet, yet over time she began to control me and the more I listened, the more she spoke, ever emboldened by her own self-importance and unerring belief that everything she said was gospel. So, when Mrs Zippy said that I should only 'eat really bland-tasting meals because rich flavours equal fat', I listened. And when Mrs Zippy said, 'Use diet pills, drink Diet Coke and smoke cigarettes to keep the weight off.' I listened. When Mrs Zippy said, 'Stay on the protein-only phase of Atkins for three years.' again I listened. Finally, when Mrs Zippy said I shouldn't get a shiny-star sticker for any of the small successes in my life, guess what? I listened.

I was really tired of allowing her to push me around and demand these crazy requests, so I called her out into the light and this worked for me for several reasons.

When I started visualising my inner negative voice as a character, it helped to foster the belief that it was separate from me and therefore I could distance myself from the hurtful things it would say. Now, all of a sudden, it felt like the nasty words weren't coming from the 'inside me' and therefore could be disregarded a little more easily.

Next, I chose an identity for it that is inherently comical. By turning mine from a sinister voice lurking in the dark into a puppet in a bright, colourful TV studio, where there was nowhere for her to hide, my puppet could no longer say mean things from the shadows. In other words, I was able to strip Mrs Zippy of her menace. Where once she had existed in the darkest recesses of my subconscious, now she was forced into the spotlight.

Now when she speaks, I see her for what she really is: a silly puppet that has no place telling me how to live my life. And because mine was based on a female version of Zippy from *Rainbow*, it meant she, also, had a zip on her mouth. So whenever she gets out of line, I hold up my hand and say 'Hey lady – you are on a warning here. If you speak to me like that again you will leave me no choice but to silence you.'

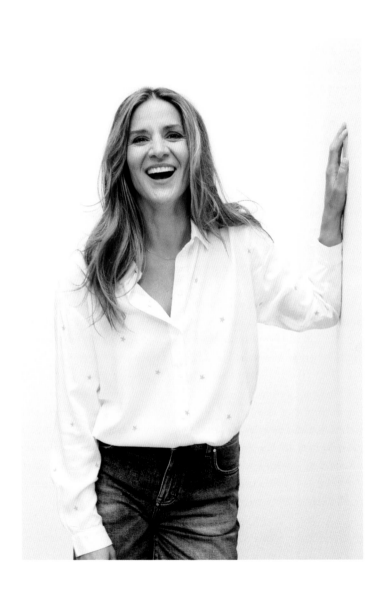

As bitchy as she is to me, I am always really careful not to be nasty back, so whenever I speak to her I am firm but fair and never lose my temper or hurl abuse. In fact, before I speak to her, I often take a deep measured breath that lasts 16 seconds and acts as what is known as a 'pattern interrupt'. It is a simple practice designed to offer a moment of pause and by filling our bodies with oxygen and our minds with silence, we can avoid rising to the triggers that often set us off. And speaking of triggers, the pattern-interrupt technique is used by US Special Forces, where clear thinking and an even temperament are literally a matter of life and death.

The technique is simple: inhale for four seconds, hold for eight seconds and exhale for four seconds. As you slowly breathe in, hold the breath and breathe out again, focus on the counting of the numbers, the swelling of your chest and the sound of the air flowing through your lungs. These 16 seconds are just a tiny fraction of time but will make a huge difference and often when your personal puppet is in full flow, this will literally starve the voice of oxygen and give you a chance to reset.

Once you have had a breath and the puppet continues to bitch, then without a hint of hesitation reach out and zip her mouth shut. She is now voiceless, mute and thus powerless. With a simple mental gesture we can reduce a bully to an object of ridicule as she struggles to unzip her mouth with her big, clownish hands.

So try it! It will seem silly at first, but that is part of the point. Now, you may choose to visualise your puppet as a more traditional type of sock puppet; like the ones you might have made as a kid. Go into as much detail as you want. Make it a dirty, unwanted partner-less sock destined for the bin, with wonky buttons for eyes and holes all over. Better still, give it a silly voice so that the next time it starts saying things like, 'You should not have eaten that' or 'You are a bad mother' you can see it for what it really is, a pathetic puppet with a silly voice that you rescued from the bin.

Whatever you choose to make it look or sound like, make sure it is definitely a puppet rather than a person, because it is important to remember that whatever shape this voice takes, *you* are the one who is in control. This puppet is an extension of you, which means you control it, not the other way around. Put simply, it is your hand up the puppet's arse making its mouth move, so make sure it knows who is the boss.

So, now that you have given your puppet an identity, you must challenge it the next time it speaks, because it is extremely likely that its view of the real world is not actually based on reality. There are two ways to challenge the puppet:

❶ Prove it wrong with facts and educate yourself so you can correct any erroneous myths your puppet is clinging on to. For years, when Mrs Zippy kept telling me the only way to have a healthy body was to deprive myself, I listened. It wasn't until I studied nutrition and fitness that I was able to confidently tell her to fuck off with her misguided 'facts'.

❷ Listen more to the outside world; believing *your ears* rather than relying on *her voice* to always guide you. A prime example of this is 'The Compliment Syndrome'.

THE COMPLIMENT SYNDROME

—

You know the drill. You are wearing your best summer frock that just cost you 100 quid, and you had saved for months to get your manicured mitts on it. You have also been feeling quite good about yourself as you have been eating well and getting plenty of rest and exercise and your skin is glowing.

It's Josephine's big summer BBQ party, and you are giving your frock (and you) the grand premiere they deserve. Not long after you arrive, the comments about how divine your dress is are flying in. And not just that, the compliments about how *you* look *in* the floral wonder are flooding in too. However, every time a compliment is thrown your way, your immediate knee-jerk reaction seems to be, 'Oh this old rag? It only cost a few quid in Top Shop' or 'Me? Christ no, I look like a haggard, fat old whale.'

When the person tries to reaffirm their feelings with, 'No, the dress is amazing and you look incredible in it!', you mutter something incomprehensible with words to this effect (in no particular order): 'Emm, noooo, mess, old, tired, rags, haggard, whale, beach.'

The chances are that you don't believe for one second that your dress is a horrid old rag or that you look like an actual whale gasping for its life on a soggy beach. After all, you put on your BBQ best and swanned into Josephine's back garden feeling rather like Beyoncé on her best day.

But somewhere along the way, someone told us that it was obnoxious to agree with positive comments, so we have become physically and emotionally allergic to external positive approvals. As a result, our inner voice has learned to swat compliments away with lightning-fast negative reactions.

The major issue with this is that as soon as we reject a positive comment with a degrading reply, we immediately imprint the negative spin into our own mind and also in that of the compliment-giver. I know people who, regardless of how they look, will always tell me they look horrible. And no matter how many times I try to express that they look great, they continue to insist that they are a complete 'mess'. So over time, I stop telling them they look well, because it is exhausting trying to convince someone that they deserve a compliment. Do you really want to be that girl? Well, me neither.

So after years of being the haggard old whale in the cheap Top Shop number, I decided to change the record and to accept the compliments instead. Now, when someone says something nice, I stop, smile and say ... 'Ah, thank you, that's such a nice thing to say, I really appreciate that.'

You are not saying, 'Yes, I agree, look at me, everyone, I am the dog's bollox,' (although, there would be absolutely nothing wrong with that at all because you ARE the dog's bollox). You are simply accepting the fact that they have paid you a beautiful compliment and you are thanking them for taking the time to do so.

I cannot tell you what a difference accepting compliments has made not only to my opinion of myself, but probably to other people's opinions of me too. Because, after a while, you begin to really believe the positives, and you will exude an invisible energy that is to be reckoned with. You will learn to always graciously agree with someone's lovely opinion of you, because let's face it, rejecting it is rejecting their point of view, and telling them that they are full of shit. That's not only embarrassing for them; it's also rude! After all, what gives us the right to tell someone else what he or she thinks?

Also, do not think that you always have to return a compliment. Sure, it's nice and it's respectful, but it is not always necessary. People do not offer compliments just to get one in return. Often it can seem disingenuous and forced and ends up feeling awkward. 'You look great', 'No, YOU look great', 'Ah but you look better'... #awks.

When you are given a compliment and Mrs Zippy pipes up and rejects it, then you can squash her by reminding her that you would rather listen to the nice thing you have just been told instead because, after all, she is just a sock on a hand that knows nothing.

If you find that when you scour the outside world for positive comments and you can't find any to challenge your puppet, then one of two things is probably happening:

❶ You aren't listening carefully enough, so the positive and uplifting comments you are receiving are going unheard.

❷ You are in an environment where positive words are not being uttered in your general direction frequently enough. If that is the case then you need to examine who you are speaking with and how you are being spoken to. We all deserve to be treated with dignity and affection and if those around you are not lifting you up, then call them out and tell them you would like to be spoken to with respect, or else ... zip it!

Hopefully, once you have found the secret to standing up to your internal sock puppet, you can use these same techniques in the face of aggressive, judgemental and negative voices in the real world.

And now dear reader, I am going to give you a compliment and an example of your new reply:

ME: 'You're awesome.'
YOU: 'Ah, thank you for saying so!'
ME: 'You're welcome!'

And they all lived awesomely ever after.

- Give your inner negative voice a body and a name (preferably a silly one).

- Know that you are in control of it, so that when it gets out of hand you can deal with it. You control everything in your mind. After all, you own your own mind.

- Challenge it. If it speaks up, tell it you know it is wrong because you are listening to the other real-life voices instead.

- Silence it. You have the power to tell it to be quiet and if it doesn't shut up, just mentally zip its mouth shut.

- Be vigilant. Because even when Mrs Zippy is in the spotlight, she can be pretty quick to pipe up when she's not wanted.

- The quickest and simplest way to stop her is to use the 16-second breathing technique to interrupt the pattern (see page 90).

- Remember to always stop before you reject a compliment – thank the giver for giving it and believe that you are worthy of the lovely things they have just said to you.

This is also reminder to speak kindly to others. We all know the power words have, which means we have a responsibility to wield them carefully. Imagine how you would feel if you were unwittingly feeding the sock puppet of a friend, family member or even a total stranger with unkind expressions, words or acts.

Finally, remember that your puppet loves the 'C' word ... no, not that one, the other one. Cynicism. It will take great pleasure from cutting things down or fobbing them off. It is an expert at taking things for granted and ignoring the magnificence of your very existence. The most effective way to combat the 'C' is with the 'G' word – gratitude.

GRATITUDE (AND WHY IT MATTERS TO YOUR OVERALL WELLBEING)

—

When my Switch moment arrived, I had started to think deeply: about how lucky we are to be here, what that actually means for the way we live our lives and how that affects our physical and mental health.

It was during a night flight, as I looked out of the tiny window at the starry sky, that I began thinking about the Universe. I think it is safe to say that, regardless of your philosophy, religion or view of how we came into existence, we can all agree that it is pretty amazing that it happened at all. In my best Professor Brian Cox voice, let me explain ...

The Universe began 13.9 billion years ago and is a really, really big place. So big that, at the last count, there were more than 200 billion galaxies, each containing billions of stars. And of all those billions if not trillions of opportunities for life to exist, as of right now, ours is the only planet in the entire Universe with the perfect conditions for life.

From here, I'll save some time and fast forward past the formation of Planet Earth (4.6 billion years ago), past the advent of single-celled organisms (3 billion years ago) scooch past the dinosaurs and arrive at the evolution of modern humans (I won't go in to the minutiae – you get the Darwin drift) and they reckon that on Planet Earth right now there are approximately 7.8 billion of us. This means you are not 'one in a million' as the expression goes, you're actually one in 7.8 billion, baby!

And what of all the other versions of you that could have been walking in your shoes? For this we are going to have to go to some pretty sticky places and by sticky, I mean really sticky because we need to talk about sperm, aka semen, spunk, jizzmundo, baby-batter. Before this gets out of hand (no pun intended) here is some semen science:

The average volume of semen produced at ejaculation is around 3ml and contained within that are about 300 million sperm cells. So conservatively speaking, if a man starts creating sperm at 15 years old and lives until he is 85, that is 70 years' worth of sperm production. In that time, let's say he has a party in his pants on average three times a week (let's be honest, it is probably a lot more than this), that's 15ml of the good stuff per week and almost 1 litre per year. Over a lifetime, that's enough to fill a hot tub (that you never want to get into) where there will be more sperm cells than there are grains of sand in all the world's deserts and even stars in the night sky.

Now consider this hot tub has not been filled by just the average guy on the street but your dear old dad. Sorry, people – that's life. Now remember each of these cells is a slightly different arrangement of Dad's DNA, which means the chances of you being you are ridiculously remote. In fact, since the very moment you were conceived you were already defying odds of trillions and billions and millions to one! And that is without taking into account all the eggs that left your mum's ovaries only to find the dance hall empty when they showed up for their big date. In short, YOU are the sperm that made it! Repeat after me: 'I am so fucking lucky to be here!'

So now we know how lucky we are to be here, what does that mean in *practical terms* and how powerful a tool is a daily gratitude practice as you journey towards a healthier and happier you? Well, the answer is, very powerful indeed!

THE LIMESCALE OF NEGATIVITY

I compare the tough, old nasty negativity that takes the shine away from life and makes everything look lifeless, dull and grey, to limescale. And I compare gratitude to a limescale remover that smells of lemon zest and offers the promise of a cartoon sparkle as it gets rid of the hard, crusty, gritty layer that accumulates around the showerhead, taps and generally hard-to-reach areas.

Just like limescale, negativity builds up easily and gets tougher to remove the longer you leave it. It is stuck in every conceivable crevice and so engrained that it is really hard to shift in just one cleanout. This bugger needs to be removed with some regular elbow grease and the simple solution is equivalent to a daily practice of gratitude. Gratitude slowly chips away at negativity and when it finally does remove it all, everything is clear, sparkling and runs so much more smoothly.

THE SHOWER OF GRATITUDE

And speaking of showers, that is exactly where I like to practise my gratitude. It might seem like a strange place to celebrate life, but bare with me (pardon the pun) and you'll see why. Firstly, I shower at least once a day, which means every day without fail I have a perfect opportunity to get into the gratitude groove. Also because I am by myself in there (unless my husband hijacks my me-time) it is a great time for self-reflection. Under the warm water I'm effectively in a mini spa, an oasis that is disconnected from my mobile, emails, social media and the big wide world. Right there in that space, I have no excuses but to be present in the moment.

So during this time I start by thinking how grateful I am for the hot water as it cascades down, knowing that there are so many people who do not have access to this luxury we take for granted. Next, I think about the boiler that makes this water nice and toasty and I am grateful for the fact that it is there, chugging away in the background seven days a week, making sure there is always warm water for me whenever I want it. It's funny that the only time we really notice our boiler is when it breaks down and yet even then, if it does pack up, we have a phone to connect us to a specialist who comes directly to our door to fix it.

I think about the other things in my home too, such as the electricity that powers the lights, dishwasher and WiFi, all at the flick of a switch. I think about the internet and my laptop that affords me instant video calling to speak to my best friend in Sydney or my parents in Dublin. Even though the ones we love are sometimes hundreds or even thousands of miles away, we can still have them with us in the room as though they are right by our side. Having my parents close is so important to me and I feel grateful that they nurtured me, raised me with praise and support, educated me and told me it was always OK to take the path that made me the happiest.

Now, this is the fun part because once I am holding all of the things that I am most grateful for in my mind's eye, I suddenly switch the shower to freezing cold! Holy shit! The icy water runs down my spine, takes my breath away and reminds me that YES! I AM ALIVE! This practice will wake your brain up, get your immune system going and make you realise how alive you are. Aim for 10 seconds to begin with and work your way up to a minute. Give it a go – it will set you up for the day!

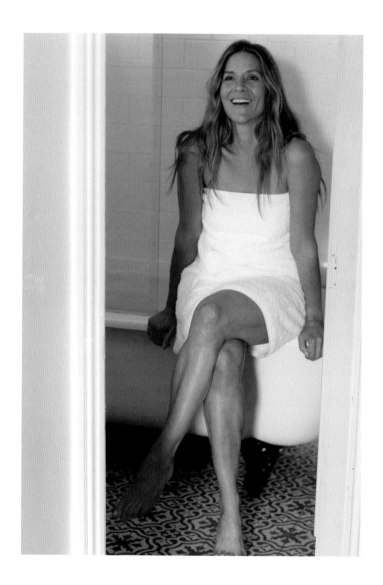

AMAZING GRACE

Another way to be grateful is to be outspoken. Get into a habit of saying *out loud* that you are thankful and you will find that you are more at peace with yourself and the world around you. A good way to practise out-loud gratitude is to start saying grace at mealtimes. You don't have to be religious and it doesn't matter if you are thanking God, Allah, Buddha or Ronald McDonald, it's just nice to take a moment to say how grateful you are for the food you have in front of you.

REASONS TO BE GRATEFUL

❶ You are completely unique.

❷ No odds are insurmountable in the face of what you have already achieved just to be here.

❸ You are so fortunate to be on this planet, so don't waste your life sweating the small stuff.

❹ Your dad is a serious spunk machine.

⟶ SWITCH TIPS ⟵

- Negativity is like limescale; use gratitude practices daily to stop it building up.

- Every day when you shower, take time to be thankful for the things in your life.

- Turn on the cold tap for 10 seconds at the end of your shower; it is a great way of centering your focus and reminding you how good you have it.

- Be inclusive and encourage gratitude in others. For example, say grace with your kids or a little prayer at night before they go to bed.

- Be outspoken! Get into a habit of saying *out loud* that you are thankful and you will find that you are more at peace with yourself and the world around you:

  - 'I am grateful for my eyes so that I can read this sentence!'
  - 'I am grateful for access to healthy knowledge about my body!'
  - 'I am grateful for my awesome mattress and duvet that keep me comfy and warm at night!'

SWITCHING OUT NEGATIVE TERMINOLOGY

—

We have become so accustomed to using negative terms in our everyday vocabulary that they have become woven into the tapestry of our daily language. To reset this mindset, we need to start unpicking them with a small needle and swapping them with language that is not negative or destructive. For example, have you ever used any of the following phrases?

- Fuck my life (FML)
- Cheat day/cheat meal
- Naughty/bad foods
- Guilty pleasure

With phrases like these in common parlance, is it any wonder that we feel down and low about life sometimes and feel such a sense of shame and guilt around food? Switching out negative words for more positive alternatives will help you to be mindful and think of alternative phrases. Let's tackle them one at a time.

FUCK MY LIFE (FML)

Why? Why would you want to fuck your miraculous life and throw it under the bus? I hear people say this when nothing bad has really happened, because they have just become so accustomed to saying it. Such as when (First-World problem alert) they miss the bus, get yoghurt on their blouse, spill their chia seeds all over the kitchen or have slow WiFi. This constant repetition of saying that you want to fuck your life, even if uttered in jest, will ultimately have a subliminal effect. It will start to make you anxious, irritated and even lead to depressive feelings.

CHEAT DAY/CHEAT MEAL

There is nothing positive about the word 'cheat'. It has a very severe connotation and alludes to the fact that you have broken someone's trust or been dishonest or unfair. To associate a meal or a day with this word is so counter-productive and the complete opposite of the reason you have set out to have this meal or this day in the first place – to treat yourself because you deserve it! Swap the word 'cheat' to 'treat'. 'This is a meal/day that I am treating myself to, because I have trained hard all week, and I have eaten well to nourish my body, so I deserve this.'

NAUGHTY/BAD FOODS

Some foods are less healthy than others, but calling them 'naughty' or 'bad' is destructive. Inevitably, if you do end up eating something 'bad', then *you* in turn feel 'bad' for eating it. So replace calling 'bad' or 'naughty' foods with 'limited' foods. 'I am not going to eat too many of these, because I know that they are limited in the amount I can have before they become unhealthy.'

GUILTY PLEASURE

Guilt is an extremely negative emotion, and one that we should be avoiding at all costs. Pleasure, on the other hand, is extremely positive, and an emotion we should be drawn to. When you use the words 'guilty' and 'pleasure' together, you negate any good around the pleasurable feeling. There should never be any guilt around pleasure. Pleasurable food or activities are pleasurable, and you deserve them. Remove the word 'guilt' from all things related to food, body or activity.

THE 'BUT/AND' SCENARIO

—

Try to switch out the word 'but' for 'and' whenever you can. It will feel pretty awkward at times, and the more you practise it (it was tempting to write; 'but the more you practise it') the easier it becomes. You will find that in no time, you will sound and feel much more positive about everything. Here are some examples:

Old: 'I love your shirt *but* I think that you could change your shoes.'

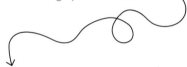

New: 'I love your shirt *and* I think that you could change your shoes, because their colour would match your shirt much better.'

Old: 'I have had the most incredible day, *but* the traffic on the way home was a disaster.'

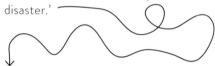

New: 'I have had the most incredible day, *and* the traffic on the way home was a disaster, so I had a chance to listen to some awesome music/a great podcast all the way home.'

In both instances the use of the word 'but' means that any words you say after the word 'but' are most likely going to sound negative. However, when you switch the 'but' for 'and', it immediately removes any negative connotation and urges the brain to process and express feelings of positivity instead.

CATASTROPHISING

—

How often have you allowed your mind to run away and imagine situations that do not end well? This is called 'catastrophising' and it happens when we make up alternate realities.

Take for example a scenario I found myself in a few years ago. I had made a suggestion about something to my agent via email. The suggestion would have meant a different deal structure with a project we were working on. I had hesitated to write it and after I wrote it I felt a slight tinge of fear as to how the email would be received, so I waited with bated breath for her reply. I did not hear back from her that day and so that evening I started to tell myself the beginning of a story that went like this: my agent had read the email, didn't like the proposal that I had made, and was stewing with fury. She had then turned to everyone else in the office and explained that I had suggested a completely ridiculous proposal. (Now, in my head, there were 10 people against me.)

She then went home to her partner and explained my ludicrous suggestion; all the while her partner was nodding their head while both of them concocted a way that I could be berated and possibly dropped from the agency. When I didn't hear from my agent the following morning, I concluded that I was indeed right and that over the weekend she was going to tell her friends and get some reinforcement before calling me on Monday to tell me that she did not want to work with me anymore.

I spent that entire weekend chewing my bottom lip with a sinking feeling in my heart, and in my head I began to plan a series of meetings with new agencies the following week. I also created several conversations with these new agents in my head with some telling me that they were too busy to represent me. Of course my self-esteem was knocked in advance, due to this imaginary scenario, and in turn my mood turned sour. I ruined experiences that weekend, because I was feeling sorry for myself; I went to watch a movie and I basically missed it because the whole way through I was thinking of how the following week was going to pan out.

Monday morning came, and I woke with a sinking feeling of impending doom that I was not in the mood to face, so I stayed in bed for an extra two hours, trying to avoid what lay ahead. The day passed without any news from my agent, which reaffirmed my suspicions. Things were not looking good. On Tuesday the phone rang, and it was her! With a defensive air, I picked up the phone, ready for what was about to come. My back was up, my answers ready, and then she hit me with it. She was calling to apologise profusely because of the delay in response – a close family friend had passed away and she had had to travel out of town for the funeral. In that moment the reality replaced the story I had told myself and I realised that I had wasted the best part of a week of my life worrying, catastrophising and beating myself up: all completely in vain.

In that moment I understood with perfect clarity the meaning of the phrase that to 'assume' something is to make an ASS out of U and ME. I vowed right there and then that no matter what happened in the future, I would always try to imagine the best-case scenario, because if I am going to tell myself a story, it might as well be a good one!

There is absolutely no point in worrying about the past because it does not exist anymore; it is simply a memory. Meanwhile, the future is 100 per cent a myth because it has not happened yet. All that you have is now.

REDEFINING DEFINITIONS AND LABELS

—

What we do, who we are, how we perceive ourselves or how we look should not define us. We humans find it so much easier to categorise each other and put each other into 'boxes', because it is safer and easier for us: our brains find it much more palatable if we can box each other off and leave it there. But labelling and defining each other and ourselves is a pastime that starts simply and can end in mental torture. Realistically, nothing should define us and we should be indefinable, yet we insist on asking the questions who am I, and what am I?

The list goes on and on and, more often than not, definitions are detrimental to our health, as they will have some form of negative connotation. This is because we are better at putting ourselves down than championing ourselves. Labels and definitions do not represent you. Your name does not even represent you. And yet, logically, the more you tell yourself you are a 'something' or a 'someone', you will not only put a limiting belief on yourself, you will also begin to believe the label, the definition and the story. This results in a loss of your 'essence'. Your essence is who you are before all the crap (the labels, the assumptions, the stories, the definitions) gets piled on top of you.

All labels and definitions are as accurate or inaccurate as you want them to be – they tell a story, a story that you make up or that someone has made up about you. And only YOU can give them reinforcement, meaning or weight. These stories allow us to make sense of life, of ourselves, of who we think we are and how we think others

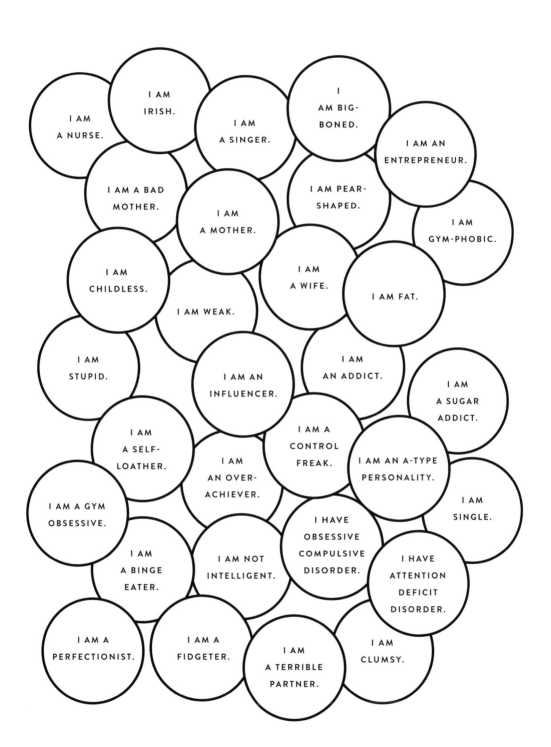

I AM A NURSE.

I AM IRISH.

I AM A SINGER.

I AM BIG-BONED.

I AM AN ENTREPRENEUR.

I AM A BAD MOTHER.

I AM A MOTHER.

I AM PEAR-SHAPED.

I AM GYM-PHOBIC.

I AM CHILDLESS.

I AM A WIFE.

I AM FAT.

I AM WEAK.

I AM STUPID.

I AM AN INFLUENCER.

I AM AN ADDICT.

I AM A SUGAR ADDICT.

I AM A SELF-LOATHER.

I AM AN OVER-ACHIEVER.

I AM A CONTROL FREAK.

I AM AN A-TYPE PERSONALITY.

I AM SINGLE.

I AM A GYM OBSESSIVE.

I AM A BINGE EATER.

I AM NOT INTELLIGENT.

I HAVE OBSESSIVE COMPULSIVE DISORDER.

I HAVE ATTENTION DEFICIT DISORDER.

I AM A PERFECTIONIST.

I AM A FIDGETER.

I AM A TERRIBLE PARTNER.

I AM CLUMSY.

perceive us. But none of it is tangible – they are all just words, and to break the habit of using these words you simply need to take a split second, ask yourself what the truth is and think of the words before they leave your mouth.

For example, the next time you are about to tell a group of friends:

• 'GOSH, I AM SO CLUMSY.'

  Stop, take a breath, and change the words to:

  'I fell over yesterday – it was an embarrassing tumble, and I recovered like a champion.'

• 'UGH! I AM SO FAT RIGHT NOW.'

  Stop, take a breath, and change the words to:

  'I am feeling a little out of shape at the moment and so I can't wait to get back into the gym this week so I can smash out some workouts like a warrior.'

• 'I WAS SUCH AN IDIOT WITH MY HUSBAND YESTERDAY, I WOULD HAVE DIVORCED MYSELF IF I COULD.'

  Stop, take a breath, and change the words to:

  'I had a little bit of an emotional stumble yesterday, and I was vulnerable in front of my husband. I am glad, though, because I was true to myself.'

• 'I AM SUCH A BAD MOTHER.'

  Stop, take a breath, and change the words to:

  'Motherhood is challenging today, but you know what? I am doing the very best I can.'

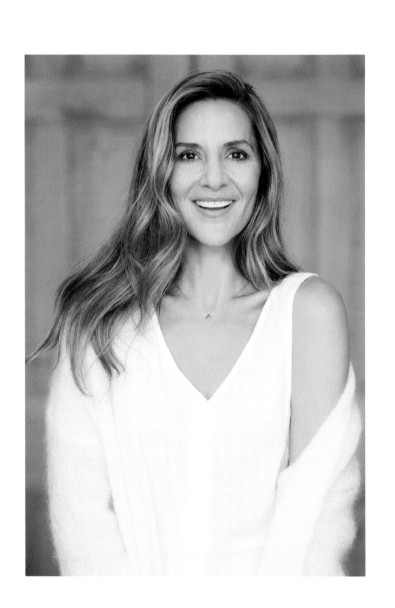

- **'I AM SO HYPER-CRITICAL OF MYSELF; I HAVE AN ISSUE WITH SELF-LOATHING.'**

  Stop, take a breath, and change the words to:

  'I know I give myself a hard time sometimes, and I don't know why, because the truth is, I am pretty awesome.'

You may often hear yourself or others say the words:

- 'I was just born like that.'
- 'That's just who I am.'
- 'I've been like this my whole life and it's worked out just fine.'
- 'I will never change now, I have been like this forever.'

Yet again, these are just the stories you tell yourself. Everything you think in life and everything you do is born out of habit. And habit is a direct result of doing the same thing over and over again. Practise anything long and hard enough and you will be able to do it without thinking.

If you can ride a bike or drive a car, can you even recall the days when you could not drive or ride a bike? I bet you don't think twice now before you buckle up behind the wheel to go and get the shopping, or sit on your saddle and push off? Well, your thought processes work in exactly the same way!

So, what does this mean? It means BINGO, babies! The nut is cracked, you CAN change, you CAN think different thoughts, you CAN speak kindly to yourself, you CAN love who you are, you CAN congratulate yourself!

Because the more you practise redefining the words that come out of your mouth (or stay in your head), the more the old way of saying these words CAN become null and void and eventually you will begin to believe the new words that you say:

- 'I am becoming a champion and a warrior.'
- 'I was being vulnerable because that was the right thing to do.'

- 'I am a really competent mother who tries so hard every day to do the right thing by my children.'
- 'I want to make a change, so I will. I understand that I can become a better version of myself, so I will be patient and take it day by day.'

By nature, we run away from change because we fear what others will think, yet the truth is that no one else matters except you. Start speaking kindly to yourself, and let others worry about what they think and what they want to believe.

Right now, I want you to ditch the definitions you have of yourself and also of those around you. You won't drop dead, you won't pass out – you might just come to life! And don't pay any heed to how others define you; just remember, what other people think of you is really none of your business. When you adopt this attitude, you will be surprised at the number of things in your life that will start to fall into place.

→ **SWITCH TIPS** ←

- Use NLP (see page 84) to change how you speak to yourself. Switch your old, usual narrative with a new one, for example switch 'Wherever I go, I don't feel like I fit in' to 'Wherever I go, I stand out.'

- Eradicate negative terminology from your vocabulary. Play a game with yourself by trying to change anything negative to positive. It's fun!

- Change the word 'but' to 'and' – you will find this tiny word switch will make huge differences to how you see things.

- Stop defining yourself. You are not defined by your name, your occupation, your marital status, your health, or anything else.

- Stop making up alternate realities! Catastrophising means that you are not focused on the present moment.

'SOMEWHERE ALONG THE WAY, WE SWALLOWED THE MESSAGE THAT "PERFECT IS BEST", A MESSAGE THAT HAS BEEN SPOON-FED TO US VIA NEWSPAPERS, MOVIES, SOCIAL MEDIA, TV SHOWS, THE WORLD WIDE WEB, MAGAZINES, POSTERS AND BILLBOARDS.'

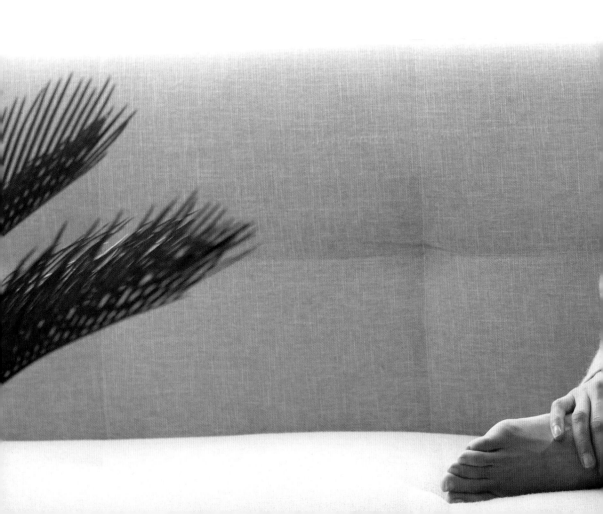

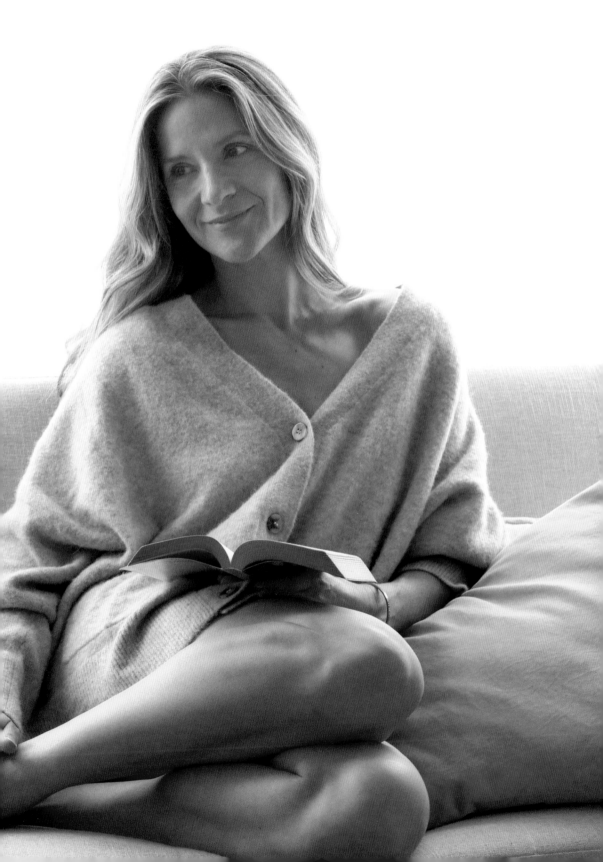

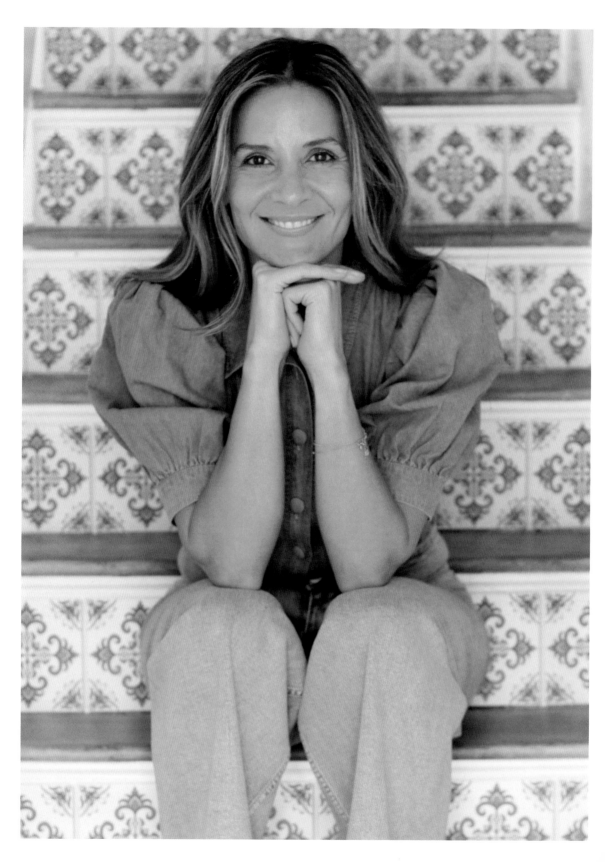

THE
PERFECTION
TREADMILL

$\longleftrightarrow$

FOR SOME REASON, we women feel the need to be the most perfect versions of ourselves, in every single way. We strive every day to be the very best at everything: the perfect mother (insert your own school gate war here), daughter, partner, sister and friend. We want to be the strongest women (I can lift these bags and these two babies all by myself: cue chiropractor sessions for a year), the least needy women (see previous example) and the ones most capable of thriving without help (you get the drift). And to pop the unglazed cherry on top of the sugar-free icing, we want the perfect body to visibly show just how fucking perfect we are.

We are driven towards this desire so badly that we not only physically drive ourselves to exhaustion, we also batter ourselves mentally, often believing that if we have not yet reached a stage of perfection, nothing else will do. And so we try and try and try until we succeed – except perfection does not exist, so we just keep trying.

So just why have we become so obsessed with this idea of 'perfect'? Somewhere along the way, we swallowed the message that 'perfect is best', a message that has been spoon-fed to us via newspapers, movies, social media, TV shows, the World Wide Web, magazines, posters and billboards. Without us realising it, this subliminal toxic messaging has been slowly seeping into our bloodstream for decades.

But the source of this toxic information is simply the food and so not entirely to blame. Our hunger for perfection lies deep within us; it has been festering in the darkest recesses of our minds for decades, ever since we were very little. And so, before we can excrete the shit we have been fed, we need to dig a little bit deeper to understand more about what perfectionism is and how we can work towards eliminating these tendencies once and for all, so that eventually – no matter how many times the 'perfect' message is shoved down our throat – we have the ability to spit it out.

'Perfect' is a word we seem to dine out on on a regular basis. It is a word that we bandy about proudly like it's the best thing to happen since almond milk, and we just love to regale tales of being a 'perfectionist', so much so that if we had our way, we would stitch a large superwoman-style 'P' onto our H&M vest tops. I used to love calling myself a 'perfectionist', 'a control freak', 'a high achiever', remark that I had 'OCD tendencies' or proclaim with pride that I had a 'type-A personality'.

And yet it turns out that these were not exactly the fabulous monikers I thought they were. Perfectionism is defined as 'a personality disposition characterised by striving for flawlessness and setting exceedingly high standards of performance accompanied by overly critical evaluations'. Suddenly it doesn't seem quite so appealing, does it?

THE MULTIDIMENSIONAL PERFECTIONISM SCALE

—

Around the same time that Brad Pitt was making his big screen debut with Thelma and her mate Louise, Julia Roberts and Richard Gere were glamorising prostitution in *Pretty Woman* and Maggie Thatcher was hanging up her iron hat, some clever fellas named Hewitt and Flett were creating the 'Multidimensional Perfectionism Scale'. As sci-fi as this scale sounds, it's pretty grounded in (an unfortunate) reality and is very relevant to mental health today. The scale revealed that there are three types of perfectionism: self-oriented, other-oriented and socially prescribed.

SELF-ORIENTED PERFECTIONISTS

These people set themselves extremely high standards and goals – both in work and in relationships. If they lose out to a competitor, don't get a bonus at work or the job they want, fail a test or fail within a relationship, they can often feel anxiety. Because they expect to be perfect and strive to be perfect, they will always be highly self-critical if they fail.

Personally, I have set myself really high goals in both my work and relationships in the past and I always believed that this was a good thing. I thought that it set me apart from everyone else and that unless I set high goals, I would never amount to anything. I have been successful in my life, and maybe an element of this perceived perfection that I set as my benchmark was the reason for my successes. On the other hand, perhaps because I am naturally determined, I would have achieved the same result regardless.

A great example I can share with you is from a period in my life when everything crumbled around me because I did not live up to my expectation of being 'perfect' or having the 'perfect life' I so craved. I was 38, and had recently become engaged to a lovely man. Before we met, I was constantly worried that I would be left alone, 'on the shelf' with an army of cats by my side. This anxiety had sprung up because society had me believe that the image of 'normality' and 'tradition' is that of fairytales that end in 'happily ever after', not a future filled with cats and shelves.

You know the fairytale where the dashing knight in shining armour rescues us on his white horse? Where he sweeps us from 'the shelf', all the while fighting off the cats with his man sword? The fairytale where fireworks explode as he crashes through the front window on his horse with me, bedraggled and shocked on the back, past all the neighbours, who are wondering why there is a horse on my lawn and all my cats have been massacred? The fairytale where the music plays and the credits roll? You know, the bullshit fairytale that does not exist?

Yet we were brought up as little girls believing that these fairytales (well, maybe not the part about the massacred cats) are the stuff dreams are made of, and unless you are 'saved', 'swept', 'wooed' or 'romanced', then you are not aiming high enough. And unfortunately I bought it … well, almost.

I was wooed and romanced yet could not see that he was not the right guy for me. Even when he proposed, I accepted because the bellows of my deep-rooted desires to be one half of a couple, to be a wife, to have a future husband, to be engaged to be married, were louder than the tiny voice somewhere in the background that kept saying, 'Bad idea, sister, something ain't quite right.'

And so I went ahead and I planned the perfect wedding in a perfect château in the South of France, under a perfectly blossoming tree littered with twinkling tea lights shining a light on my perfect day. There was a delightfully small group of great people invited; the perfect mix. Some were coming from LA, others from Australia and the rest from the UK and Ireland. Everyone had paid the price of their tickets and I was about to pay the price of ... perfection.

A month before the wedding, I began to understand the true meaning of the word 'integrity' and how difficult a path it is to tread. I had to consider what was best for me and no one else. Not the man whose heart I was about to break, not my family who I feared I was letting down, not the friends who had spent hundreds on a two-week trip to Europe, not the château staff who had prepared the wedding of the century. Because, as my parents so wisely advised me at the time: 'A wedding is a day, a marriage is for life, and that is a long time to regret it.'

And so, I closed my eyes, I gritted my teeth, I took a deep breath and I pulled the plug. With my eyes still squeezed shut, I waited for everyone to hate me, for my friends to turn their backs on me, for the world to stop spinning on its axis and for everyone to cement the fact that I was not perfect.

However, when I opened my eyes again, the world was still spinning, my family and friends held me tight, and my fiancé, while devastated, accepted that he didn't want to be married to a woman who did not want to be his wife. Aeroplane tickets were refunded, some friends came anyway and we cried and laughed and cried some more. The château didn't implode, the dress got sold and I was left relieved.

However, the relief didn't last long and I was not prepared for what came next. The flood of emotions that followed were eventually diagnosed as depression, and not because I had cancelled the wedding, because that was the bravest and best decision I had ever made in my life. No, the depression came because I began to feel like a failure, incapable of achieving society's fairytale. I began to wonder if my chance at a perfect future had disappeared in a perfect puff of smoke.

My feelings of anxiety and depression were borne out of my incessant need to be 100 per cent at all times. I kept repeating the term 'should': 'I should have known better', 'I should have been more diligent', 'I should have handled things differently', 'I should be married by now'.

But who is telling us we 'should' be anything? We get to decide for ourselves. The point is that my idea of what 'should' have been had been shoved down my neck since I was a little girl and it was time to break free from the shoulda, woulda, coulda cycle.

Eventually, I found peace in being alone. I had reached a place where I knew that 'perfect' was an illusion and that my own expectations of myself and my life were so unrealistic that I would never be happy if I continued to look for them. By the time Julian, my husband, walked into my life, I'd come to understand that I did not have to lower my expectations to find love; instead I freed myself of expectations altogether! The happiness didn't come because he saved me or because he married me or because he rode in on his white horse or because there were fireworks or because there was a perfect meeting, or a perfect proposal or a perfect ring. It came because I stopped making up stories about what he *should* or *should not* be doing, and instead we made up our own rules ... together.

What I am saying is that I stopped looking for the perfect life, and in turn my life happened. Ultimately, life is what you make it and neither a piece of paper nor a gold band around your finger can tie you together. For the record, neither of us wears our ring, because they do not, nor should they, define our marital status. These things are symbols, and symbols mean nothing unless you yourself do the hard work at home, in your head or in your relationship.

My version of a happy ending happens every day because I now make each day end happily. Not because there is a formula, but because there isn't one. You can make it whatever you want it to be – there is no such thing as the 'norm'. *You are your own norm; you are your own perfect.*

OTHER-ORIENTED PERFECTIONISTS

These perfectionists believe that people *around* them should be perfect and hold everyone to unrealistically high standards. They are highly critical of others who fail to meet these expectations, so it's understandable that this form of perfectionism can risk needless confrontation and problems within relationships.

I can also identify with this form of perfectionism, because I used to set myself such high standards, and in turn expected those around me to march to the perfect beat of my perfect drum. However, just because my expectations of myself were high, I did not have the right to expect the same of others.

When others stepped out of line and my drum was still beating, I would get frustrated and anxious and sometimes I fell out with people. My view was that I worked hard at my job and aimed to do the very best I could, so was it too much to expect the same of everyone around me too? To me that seemed like a logical, rational and frankly simple ask. Consequently, I became frustrated at many people who got things consistently wrong, did not come up to scratch or did not meet my high standards. Looking back, I know that I should have freed myself of any expectations and understood that they were doing the very best they could do, given the task in front of them. Perhaps my drum was not being played in tune to *their* liking.

Have you ever been in a taxi and it's clear the driver hasn't got a clue where he is going? Have you felt a hint of irritation followed by blood boiling up to your brow, as you explain through gritted teeth that he is going around in circles? Have you then relayed that story to your friends and cried, 'HE HAD **ONE** JOB, **ONE** FUCKING JOB! Well, 'one job' is not necessarily true – we all have lots of jobs that we do at our own pace, to the best of our ability. If someone doesn't do something to the best of *my* ability, I have to assume they have different skillsets to me, or maybe they are not as invested in the task as I believe they should be.

If you really feel your taxi driver did not provide the service you paid for, then definitely don't give him a tip, or make a complaint and vent your frustrations that way. Alternatively, look at it like this: if he got you there safely and (almost) on time – then just let it slide and be grateful anyway.

Furthermore, it might be helpful for you to imagine that this person had just had the worst day of his life. Maybe his partner had left him that week; perhaps he had a death in the family and was not focused on the task in front of him; maybe he was given really bad news or maybe, just maybe, he was not a very good driver and probably should not have been driving you that day, or any day for that matter. And he was probably doing the very best that he was able to do – just because he didn't meet your standards, it does not mean he should be any less valued as a human being.

So give others a break and you will find that in turn you will give *yourself* a break and be less stressed and less focused on the perceived imperfections all around you.

SOCIALLY PRESCRIBED PERFECTIONISTS

These people believe that others (a parent, a boss, a child or, these days, a social media following) expect them to be perfect. They set impossibly high standards and constantly seek approval and as a result will often feel rejected or harshly scrutinised when that approval doesn't come. Consequently, their self-esteem takes a hit on a daily basis and they will ultimately experience a lot of negative emotions, guilt and shame.

I have also experienced this type of perfectionism; being in the public eye certainly does not help when it comes to feeling the need to be liked, loved or accepted. That's the name of the TV game.

But you do not have to be on TV to feel the pressure of wanting to feel loved, or not wanting to feel unloved, by those around you. A lot of socially prescribed perfectionists feel this pressure from a parent who didn't show them love or give them unconditional praise as a young child. Studies show that we form a strong sense of ourselves within the first three years of our lives and in these primary years we are extremely fragile and susceptible to external love, or indeed lack thereof.

Children need reinforcement during these years from birth to three and need to be reassured that their actions are worthy and championed. However, quite often parents are going through their own struggles, be it postnatal depression, mental health issues, a relationship breakdown, or just not being up to speed on what children need – after all, there is no true version of 'The Perfect Parent'.

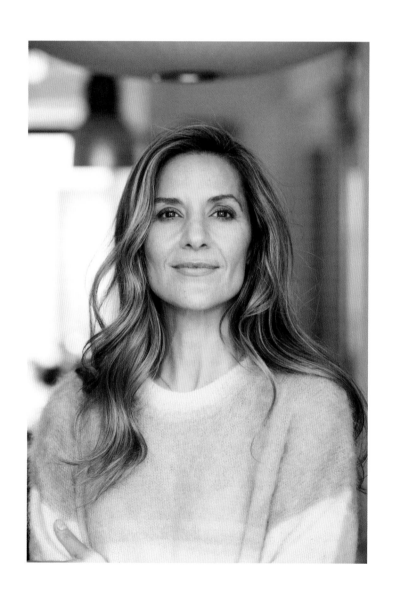

No one is perfect, not even our folks. They do the best they can do with what they've got, while being massively hormonal and sleep-deprived and, let's face it, having to learn to speak the language of goo-goo-gaga and the words to every Peppa Pig song, is enough to make anyone lose their shit. But I digress.

The point is, if you feel your parents, or others, did not lavish enough praise on you when you were younger (or even now that you are grown up), this often causes you to feel an innate need as an adult to constantly please them or others around you. It's not only in the early years that this syndrome can come into being. For example, if your parents split up when you were a teen or even an adult, you may often feel the need to take a side or to impress one or both parents. This can lead to a sense of inadequacy and as a side-effect you may feel the need to please *everyone* all the time. When we try to impress and fail, our self-esteem takes a battering and we promise ourselves that we will try better next time and when that does not happen, the cycle continues.

It is no coincidence that socially prescribed perfectionism is at an all-time high, because we now live in an age where social media has seeped into our daily consciousness like molten lava pouring over our past selves and forming new valleys of desperation, expectation and perfection.

Could it be that the steep increase of socially prescribed perfectionism is directly related to the rise of users in a social media generation? After all, we 'use' these forums as we would 'use' drugs, constantly seeking the 'high' that is our reward, in the form of likes and comments, i.e. positive reinforcement.

Studies have shown that with each 'refresh' of your screen to update the likes and comments, your brain releases dopamine (the same neurotransmitter that gets sparked when you snort a line of cocaine) and so the more likes you get, the more you continue to seek the high. This chain of events is no coincidence – it has been carefully planned by the clever bastards in Silicon Valley to manipulate your brain into thinking it is being rewarded with each shiny new 'like', 'love heart' or 'thumbs up'. 'Look, Daddy, someone hearts my photo! And look, Mummy, I got a big blue thumbs up on my bikini photo. This must mean they love me because I am perfect, right?'

Wrong.

The heart-breaking part is that when the love-hearts and thumbs-ups stop coming, we start coming down. The high spirals downwards and patterns of anxiety, shame and guilt set in. This is called a 'comedown', very similar to what you would experience in the aftermath of taking a Class A drug. So you can see, social media is in the truest sense of the word 'addictive' – mentally, physically and emotionally. It has created what we have translated into immense pressure from those around us to perform, look good, sound great and, more important, be a filtered and perfect version of ourselves. If Instagram offers you 'instant perfection' through a series of lies, filters and re-touching, then how can you ever even begin to keep up with that level of perfectionism in real life? We set ourselves up for an instant fail when we pretend our body, life, relationship or job is not what it is.

I once sat behind a couple on a plane. They had been drinking and were starting to argue. The argument got so heated at one point that they each threw a drink in the other's face, much to the mixed amusement and horror of everyone around. What was even more amusing/horrifying, though, was that as the plane came into land, the girl took out her phone and snapped a pouting selfie with her leftover G & T. As I peered through the seats, fascinated, I was flummoxed to see her posting the photo on Instagram with the caption, 'Landed. Holiday. Paradise. Perfect.' It made me realise just how sad it is that we portray a false image of perfection to the people we are supposed to be the closest to, just so we can have an archive of perfection in a web server somewhere in California.

It is when things go tits up or when you realise after you put the phone away that you are not perfect, and your boyfriend is reeling beside you on a plane with half a G & T in his hair, that you are left with feelings of imperfection and inadequacy. That girl is probably forcefully reminded of those feelings every time she goes back to her Instagram feed and sees the lie she told. In these moments, we not only feel like frauds; we are reminded of our own imperfections.

It might be a wake-up call for us all to remember that socially prescribed perfectionism is the most harmful kind because it is linked with suicide, hopelessness and disordered eating and studies have shown that those with eating disorders, anxiety disorders, obsessive-compulsive disorder and depression had higher levels of perfectionism compared with people who didn't have any of the conditions.

If you feel that you might be running on the perfection treadmill, it's time to flick The Switch and get off. Here's how.

STOPPING THE PERFECTION TREADMILL: HOW TO GET OFF

FREE YOURSELF FROM EXPECTATION

Rather than lowering your expectations, which to a perfectionist can be viewed as failure in itself, the key to getting off the perfection treadmill is to free yourself from expectation altogether. After all, if we expect perfect then anything short of that unachievable mirage will always be seen as a disappointment. We can't predict the future, so the likelihood of expectations being accurate are slim, meaning that most of the time, the perfectionist is left to pick up the pieces of the inconsistencies between the fantasy of perfection and reality of a chaotic, unpredictable and dynamic world.

If we are the authors of our own stories, then why create a fiction that will almost always differ from the fact, leaving us frustrated with the results? This is true for all types of perfectionist behaviours and so often, an expectation of how something 'should be' can ruin what could be a joyous occasion. For me the classic example of misplaced expectations is the 'Airport Collection Conundrum'.

She and He are the 'perfect couple'. Both are high achievers, go-getters and live by the perfectionist's mantra, 'I expect a lot from the people around me and even more from myself.' They have been dating for a while and things are starting to get serious. She went away on a work trip for a week to New York City and on her return He wants to make an impression so he offers to collect her from the airport. The flight lands at 6.40 a.m. So far, so good, but thanks to 'expectation', this is where things start to go wrong. Because on the way to the airport he creates a scene in his mind where she steps off the plane looking like a movie star who showers him with affection and gratitude for waking up at 4 a.m. to brave the motorway.

Meanwhile, She pictures a scene where her handsome prince is waiting eagerly with a bunch of peonies (her favourite) and she runs towards him passionately as he picks her up and performs Swayze's *Dirty Dancing* finale move, just as 'The Time Of My Life' blares over the airport tannoy. But as She exits the gate feeling bleary-eyed and bloated, she cannot see His face in the crowd. Surely there is some mistake, or He must be perfecting his Swayze move in the bathroom. When She texts him, He explains that he is outside waiting at the drop-off point and to please hurry as he is being eyed up by airport security. When She arrives at the car (internally seething), the engine still running and exhaust fumes billowing into her face as she coughs and splutters, He emerges, disappointed not to see the glamour puss he was so hotly anticipating, instead a coughing mess who looks slightly fierce and bullish. She didn't emerge from the terminal red-carpet ready, and She is not lavishing Him with praise — what the actual F?

This is an all-too-familiar occurrence that is born from a series of unrealistic expectations. What should have been a happy reunion turns into a tense car journey with both feeling annoyed at their own perceived failure and a sense of injustice. If they had just accepted that life is not scripted, it's often messy and the intention is more important than the outcome — then life would be so much simpler.

STOP SEEKING APPROVAL

Seeking approval that is not forthcoming is always going to be a fruitless exercise. I mean, if you have to force approval out of someone that is not genuine, is that really going to make you happy? It is ultimately YOU who has control over your own thoughts, so if you choose to feel inadequate you will feel inadequate; if you choose to feel that your actions are valid, celebrating all the micro-wins along the way, you will feel comforted and sleep better at night.

RID YOURSELF OF THE STIGMA

If you happen to have grown up with a parent who was not present emotionally or physically, be mindful not to wear this as a heavy cloak that weighs you down. It is not uncommon to interpret a parent's or caregiver's missteps as the reason for one's own anxiety or behaviours. While these things are definitely valid, and need to be worked on between parties, the key here is not to imprison yourself in a jail that someone else made. Break free of others, past misdoings, personality traits or actions. Rid yourself of other people's labels and become your own version of yourself.

DELETE INSTAGRAM

Many of us using social media assume that we are not good enough if our 'followers' or 'fans' did not 'like' our latest post or if someone makes a comment that is displeasing, negative or hurtful. Why constantly choose to torture yourself by choice? If you feel as though this little app is making you feel insignificant or giving you feelings of inadequacy, delete it from your phone. If this is something you are not ready to do, then go to the next step.

INSTA-HACKS

Stop looking at your phone first thing in the morning. Is the first thing you want to see when you wake up someone else's life, the party you were not invited to, the boyfriend you don't have or the holiday you're not on? Without knowing it, you just started your day with a sense of jealousy, dislike, injustice, seething and inadequacy and you have theoretically put your grumpy boots on and set off on your journey to work. All day these feelings will bubble away under the surface of your skin, and you may not even be aware of them. You go to bed looking at social media, an act that confirms the feelings you woke up to, and you will probably have nightmares about the designer bag you are not rocking, the six pack you are not packing and the hot man who is snogging your teenage nemesis, not you. Day after day, evening after evening you layer these feelings on top of each other. So take control with simple tricks like charging your phone overnight in another room and only go to it after you have woken up, showered (complete with gratitude practice, page 95) and are ready for the day. This will ensure that you have already set your mood, which is a good one, and nothing, not even your teenage nemesis's hot man, can get in your way.

HAVE EMPATHY

If you feel someone has fallen short of your high standards, then review why you are imposing these false levels on them by empathising. Ask yourself, what are they going through? What's happening in their lives? Why did they fall short and why am I putting so much emphasis on someone else's doing, achievements or lack thereof? I can only control my own thoughts, feelings and actions and if their perceived failure has ramifications for me then I need to understand why it impacts me. If I feel like someone at work did not pull his or her weight, and in turn the pitch was not good enough and as a result I didn't get the account or the promotion – then I need to assess my own part in the whole thing.

Let me leave you with this little exercise. Close your eyes and start imagining yourself in the sea. You are on a bright and colourful unicorn lilo, that looks the part and it is safe and buoyant ... to begin with. You look outwards and see the 'perfect' horizon. This is your destination because there everything looks beautiful, clear and, well ... perfect. But soon you realise that the horizon just keeps getting further and further away and no matter how hard you paddle, you can't seem to get any closer. You become more and more exhausted. By the time you finally realise the horizon is out of reach, your lilo has been compromised: it has lost some air, and it's slowly starting to sink. You turn round and see the shore, but you are too far out now and you still really want to get to the horizon. When your unicorn lilo finally bursts, you realise that you are in deep water and are now out of your depth. The only way home is to be rescued by the realisation that you can't ever get to the horizon, so now you need to turn back and use all your energy to get to safe land. The perfect horizon was just an illusion; a place you created in your mind.

Remember, perfectionism is not something to be proud of and perfectionists take less pleasure from success than other people do. Since it has also been linked with suicide it is time to look deep within and stop reaching for the elusive 'perfect' – pronto.

→ **SWITCH TIPS** ←

- Free yourself from expectation. If you are the author of your own story, why not write one that is free of expectations? Enjoy the outcome, no matter what.

- It is all too easy to use others' actions towards us as an excuse for our own actions or behaviour. In your mind's eye, take off the heavy cloak. Now you can become your own version of you.

- Seeking constant approval is dangerous. Throw caution to the wind and let it go; you are brilliant just as you are, regardless of others' approval. Start pleasing yourself. You will find it very liberating.

- Get away from social media. Silence it, take it off your phone, limit your time spent on it. YOU have the power to do that. Only look at your phone after you have woken up and after you have reminded yourself what you are grateful for. If you *still* feel the need to look at it, then at least you will do so with grateful eyes and a strong mind.

- Give others a break. Try to put yourself in their shoes and imagine that they might be suffering. Always be kind.

'THESE GOOD HABITS WILL REPLACE THE BAD ONES THAT USED TO DOMINATE YOUR DAYS. ONCE THAT HAPPENS, YOU WILL HAVE SUCCESSFULLY FORGED A NEW LIFESTYLE THAT INCORPORATES YOUR IMPROVED WAY OF THINKING.'

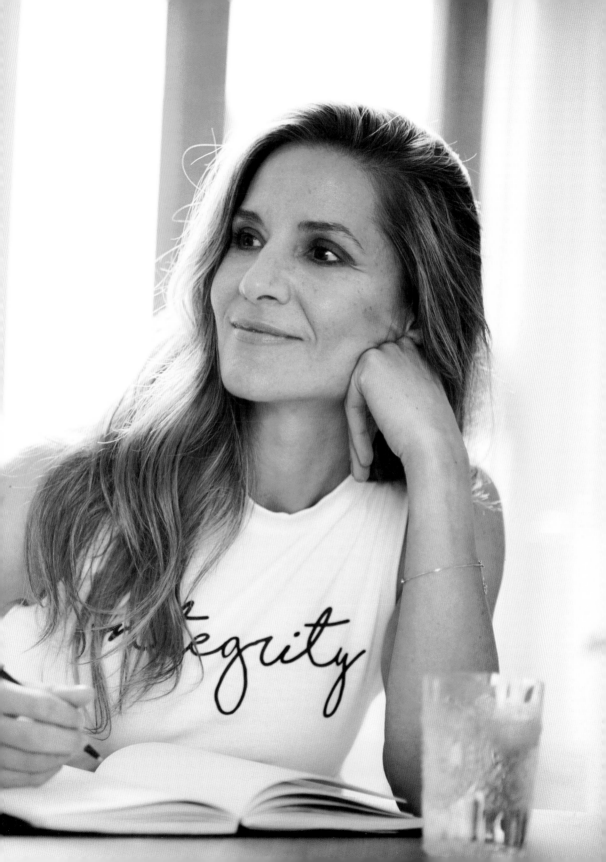

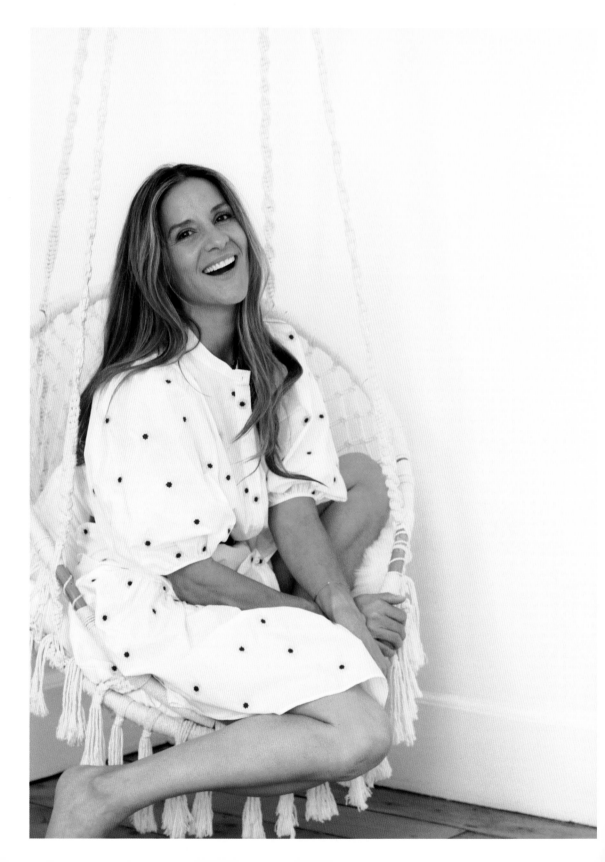

THE ART* OF
CONSCIOUS
GOAL-SETTING

*It's not an art — it's more of a science!

SOMETIMES, SIMPLY THE THOUGHT of goal-setting can seem exhausting, especially if you have tried to set goals in the past and it hasn't gone the way you'd hoped. We've all been there. It begins with an enthusiastic yet vague promise that rapidly mutates into a self-imposed chore that can eventually be quietly forgotten about and discarded, never to be spoken of again. For example, take the absolute A1, top-of-the-pile, all-conquering king of vague goals ... the New Year's Resolution, or NYR.

THE NEW YEAR'S RESOLUTION

—

It's 8 p.m. on December 31st. You're just out of the shower having used that lovely new body scrub you got in the office Secret Santa. Excited for the night ahead, you gleefully plan your NYE celebration party outfit, yet as you catch a glimpse of yourself naked in the mirror, your entire focus shifts with laser-guided precision to all the bumps and lumps that no one else notices and you begin to regret your December dietary decisions.

The critical voice in your head reminds you that, once again, over Christmas you went too far with the booze, mince pies and Cadbury's Heroes. A month-long campaign of party nights, dinners and box-set bingeing has caught up with you and as your eyes squint in disgust at your reflection, you vow that something has to change ... 'Tomorrow, the diet and exercise regime begins.' You make a wishy-washy promise about your upcoming diet that comes straight out of *The Donald Trump Bumper Book of Vague Statements*. Something like, 'This is going to be a great, great diet. The best. This diet will make a huge difference. All the other diets were losers but this is will be the best. Believe me.' Make Amanda Great Again #MAGA.

Your sock puppet hears your promise and retorts with a snarky remark, 'Fat chance, fatso!' she says, 'you'll break this get-fit promise faster than you can say high-intensity interval training.' But despite her put-downs, you know you will prove her wrong this time, so safe in the knowledge that everything will be fixed in the morning, you head out for one last night of shots, champers and seriously questionable food choices at 3 a.m.

Next morning, you wake up with an epic hangover yet despite drinking too much, sleeping too little and feeling more dehydrated than a Saharan desert sandfly, the diet and exercise plan has begun. A promise is a promise, after all. That means skip breakfast (it's 12:30 p.m. anyway) and definitely no sweet things today. You grab your trainers (hello old friends) and head out for a light jog just to ease yourself back into it. Light dinner and definitely no dessert! You wonder why you ever needed that shite in the first place!

January 2nd is a breeze. Last night you were in bed by 9 p.m. and this morning you may be a little sore, but nothing is going to stop you. A healthy breakfast is followed by another jog and along the way you delight in telling everyone that you're on your 'way to wellness'.

By January 3rd, things aren't quite as easy. Your muscles are screaming , you're starving and the winter weather is in full effect. 'Maybe today is a rest day, shouldn't overdo it ...' you declare. Meanwhile, there are still a few Christmas chocolates hanging around in the fridge, which could be thrown in the bin or ... come on, one or two can't hurt. Besides, you have been burning calories off left, right and centre, plus tonight you are planning a carb-free dinner again ... and so it goes on.

Cut to mid-January and your good intentions have melted away like Aled Jones's Snowman. And like that Snowman, you feel like you went from walking in the air to a dirty puddle of shame, doubt and resignation in just a couple of wintry weeks.

The worst part is that by breaking the deal you made with yourself, you handed your sock puppet a box full of ammo to shoot you down with by giving her the perfect example of how you can't keep a promise. Next year, why even waste the time with the middleman? You might as well look in the mirror, offer your sock puppet a megaphone and bow your head while she shouts, 'Starting tomorrow you are going to make an overblown declaration you have no intention of keeping to. When you break it I'll be waiting right here, ready to remind you that you're a big, fat liar. And speaking of fat ... you know that weight you put on over Christmas? That's your new baseline. See you next year, you dumb bitch!'

And that's the way it goes. If you were smiling knowingly at the start of that story, I hope that by the end you realised the danger of this cycle. Also consider that by the time you get into your forties you might have been making and breaking NYRs for most of your life. Unfortunately, over the years, every broken promise you made to yourself was logged in Mrs Zippy's *Giant Book of Failures*. Now, each one acts as a reminder the next time you consider stepping out in rebellion against that critical voice in your head.

Worst of all is that we don't even realise it's happening, allowing this silent and insidious behavioural pattern to grip hold of us, like an addiction to a drug we didn't even know we were taking.

Here's the good news: the cycle of broken promises and self-flagellation can be broken with deliberate, meaningful and conscious goal-setting, allowing you, once and for all, to make The Switch. With a clear plan in place as well as some grit and determination, you'll be able to stay on course long enough for these conscious daily efforts to become unconscious good habits. Moreover, these good habits will replace the bad ones that used to dominate your days. Once that happens, you will have successfully forged a new lifestyle that incorporates your improved way of thinking ... without even thinking about it. The ultimate aim is for you to no longer even consider the goal that you originally set out to achieve.

Take, for example, the ritual of brushing your teeth. Each morning you wake up, and instinctively know that you should brush your teeth before you leave the house. Similarly, before bed your routine will, 100 per cent without fail, include brushing your teeth. It wasn't always this way – as a kid I remember it being such a chore to stand there for two minutes and brush away. I would do anything to avoid it, even wet the brush and gargle some mouthwash in a bid to con my mum into believing I had brushed.

These days, of course, I could not imagine a world where I wouldn't brush, which highlights that these instructions were not pre-programmed in my DNA from birth; they were small practices that became habits which now stick to me like toothpaste on my favourite dress moments before a red-carpet event.

Brushing your teeth twice a day with no thought proves that you are already a prolific goal-setter, and there are countless more examples in your personal history where you have set a goal and then achieved it. The simple fact that you are reading these words is spectacular proof that although you were once an illiterate toddler, through planning, practising and progressing you eventually learned to convert the meaningless little squiggles on the page into words. So give yourself a high five! Interestingly, a solo high five is also known as 'clapping' but either way, you deserve it.

So where to start? Well, first you need to make the effort to actually set some goals … how many times have you thought about setting goals only for the intention to evaporate? Before you know it a few months have passed and your goal to 'set goals' has become a goal you can't seem to set!

GOALS: THE FIVE-STEP PROCESS

—

So TODAY IS THE DAY! Setting goals is a simple five-step process that can easily be remembered by using the acronym GOALS:

- **G**o!
- **O**rganise orbits
- **A**ssess, accuracy, accountability
- **L**ifestyle
- **S**mall steps

Read through all the following steps first so you fully understand the process before going back and starting in earnest. Once you're in the mood and have the time, you will need roughly two hours, so find a quiet place and grab a pen, a glass of water and a notebook. (Not *The Notebook* – although watching Ryan Gosling for 2 hours and 32 minutes is a very noble goal to set oneself.)

Before you begin, put your phone on airplane mode or, better yet, leave your mobile, laptop, iPad, iPod, pager, walkie-talkie and fax machine in another room, as this is a technology-free zone. That means no Instagram, Facebook or Netflix, texts, Snapchat, tweets, TikTok, calls or chats. Just you, your thoughts and the intention to connect to the things you really want in life.

So, in the words of the aforementioned Ryan Gosling in *The Notebook*, 'WHAT DO YOU WANT?'

GO!

Write down 28 goals as they come into your head. Splurge it, or as other authors always advised me when I was writing this book: 'puke on the page with your words'. Not the prettiest of images, but you get the drift. The main reason we write the words rather than just think or say them is because the moment you write something down, the thought, intention or goal is no longer just an abstract notion drifting around aimlessly in your head, it has now been crystallised in the real world. It exists.

List your goals in any order and don't give too much thought to what is coming out of your mind and onto the page. Although you should number them to keep track (and for another reason we'll see later on), it is important to note that the number you assign does not equal a goal's importance. For now, they are all equally valid and we'll come to how to rank and categorise them a little later.

Allow the pen to flow freely and know that the only rule here is, BE HONEST. If you are not truthful about how much you want to achieve a goal, or you don't believe in the goal, how can you ever hope to achieve it in the first place?

If nothing else, remember this simple truth when writing out your heart's desires: these are *your* goals and this is *your* journey. No one else is watching, there's no TV studio audience ready to whoop and cheer when you announce a goal you think they might want to hear. Likewise, this isn't a social media platform where you feel like you have to be the most filtered, enlightened and perfect version of yourself or the one that gets the most 'likes'. This exercise is between you, your thoughts and the paper.

So if one of your goals is to distance yourself from a friend who always upsets you, write it down. Similarly, if another is to spend more time away from your kids to work on yourself, that's OK too. After all, prioritising your happiness will ultimately benefit your family, and child protection services are not telepathically tuning in to your list, poised to accuse you of being an unfit mother.

Honesty can sometimes come with fear of judgement, so it is good to unburden yourself of this fear. No one is judging you and, just in case you need reminding, Mrs Zippy and her negative mates are most definitely not on the guest list for this particular party. So cross your arms, puff out your chest and in your best bouncer voice tell her how it is – 'Sorry, darlin', you're not on the list, so you ain't coming in.' The last thing honest and heartfelt goal-setting needs is a litany of cynical comments on what she thinks you should or should not be doing. I'll say it again … judgements are not welcome here.

So once you have written down and numbered your 28 goals, take a moment to congratulate yourself for coming this far. Life is too short not to celebrate the small wins, girls. Besides, setting your intentions in the way you just did took courage, focus, integrity and probably the most ink you have committed to paper since your last teenage break-up letter. Now take a breath, have a sip of water and get ready for the next step.

You have 28 goals randomly written out, so now it is time to examine what areas of your life these goals pertain to, and which goals deserve the most attention. To do this you'll need to pack your spacesuit, helmet and oxygen tank, then step into the command module of a rocket bound for the stars because you are about to head into orbit, baby.

ORGANISE ORBITS

When we think about our complex and multi-faceted lives it is so easy to talk about them in terms of spinning plates, yet for me the idea of plate-spinning conjures up an image of a frantic performer dashing from plate to plate, always inches away from disaster. I think it would be much nicer if we all pictured ourselves as a beautiful planet encircled by a host of different moons which all move around us gently in carefully choreographed lunar orbits.

Now just like the Earth and its lunar companion, the Moon, what happens *up there* can affect what happens *down here* – anyone else go crazy on a full moon or is it just me and the other werewolves? And that is just with one moon because 'Planet You' has seven moons, comprising:

1. Money Moon
2. Love Moon
3. Family Moon
4. Friendship Moon
5. Body Moon
6. Fun Moon
7. Mind Moon

Each of these moons will require your attention as they wax and wane through their different phases such as full moon, half moon and ... wait for it ... total eclipse! Some of your moons may orbit much closer to your planet's surface than others. Just know that if one of your moons gets too large, it might put other moons in shadow or block out the light on your planet's surface entirely. Similarly, if another of your moons goes completely off course, it might lead to a collision, resulting in all sorts of intergalactic upheaval. Further still, if you allow one of your moons to get too far away, then your

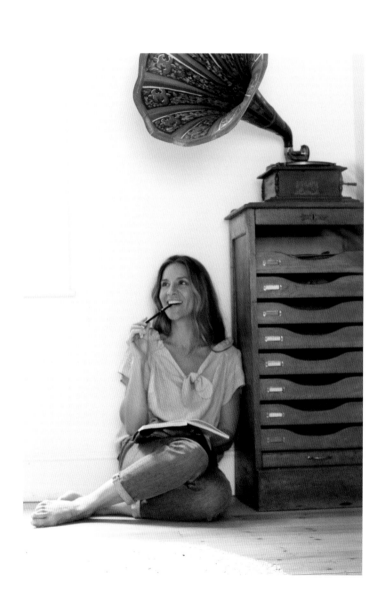

gravitational field might be too weak to hold onto it, causing it to drift off into outer space completely, and its presence will be missed.

The secret is to find a balance where each moon crosses the night sky in harmony with its sister celestial bodies: complementing rather than competing.

First you need to figure out what is personally important to you, so grab your telescope and let's look at each moon in a little more detail.

MONEY MOON

Your Money Moon is all about your relationship with cold, hard cash: everything from how you make it to how you spend it, how you save it and even how you think about it. After all, money is supposed to be a token we exchange for a better quality of life, yet so often the accumulation of money itself becomes more important than what we spend it on. A bigger bank balance does not equal a better life. That is not to say it should be wasted, squandered or completely ignored. Just know that if you let money make your world go round, you'll find yourself orbiting it, rather than it orbiting you.

This moon also includes your work life and professional satisfaction as well as the relationships you have with your colleagues. Most of us spend the majority of our time at work, so it is important to set goals pertaining to what we want from work time and where we see ourselves headed.

The Money Moon goals you set might at first look something like this:

- Make more money
- Get a promotion
- Save up for a house
- Quit my job

While they are a great start, they are going to need some work to get them to a place where we can call them *actionable blueprints for success.*

TAKEAWAY LESSON: If you let one moon make your world go round, you'll find yourself orbiting it, instead of the other way around.

We all want love, intimacy, companionship ... and someone to bleed our radiators in October — kidding (not kidding). The biggest trouble with romantic entanglements is figuring out whether you are in the right relationship or just any old relationship.

I finally figured it out the hard way. In the run up to the wedding I cancelled at 38, I remember feeling desperately unhappy, all alone and gambling with my chance to find real love yet knowing that if I didn't rip off that metaphorical emotional Band-Aid, much worse feelings would follow me the rest of my life. I was wrestling with the need to fit into a society that I imagined cared so much about my next move. Society says we 'should' be married off by a certain age, or become mothers before our eggs shrivel up and fall out of our vaginas and into the egg collection cemetery. I could not help but wonder if my swain was as good as I was going to get; if I cancelled the wedding would I be in danger of being single and childless for the rest of my life? On paper, he was 'perfect' (that word again). He was just not the right man for me.

As you know by now, finally I took the plunge and called it off. I had to be honest for both our sakes and I'm so glad I did because it paid off. Two years later, I found someone who was everything I was looking for in a life partner and much more. Had I closed myself off to that possibility I would have never found Julian, my husband, or worse still, I might have found him and caused untold damage by exploring a relationship that would have caused havoc and hurt to those around me.

So happily ever after, right? Well, yes and no because in many ways my marriage requires more work now than any of the romantic relationships that came before. Not work in a bad way because this is the person I cherish the most in the world. It is just that it can be so easy to allow neglect to set in and assume our partner will always be there no matter how we behave. That is not the case and I believe that love between lovers should not be unconditional. Making promises to each other and keeping them requires a daily commitment and often the most important relationships in our lives are the ones we take for granted or get complacent about.

Breaking unproductive patterns that have built up over time with your partner can be the hardest thing to do. That is why it is so important to set goals relating to your Love Moon so that you can consciously understand how you feel, think and behave in relationships. Think about your current partner. Do they lift you up and are they your greatest cheerleader, and more important, are you theirs? When you say to each other, 'I love you', is it true? If you don't have a partner currently, do you want one? Could it be that the relationship you need to focus on right now is the one you have with yourself?

Use this goal-setting session as an opportunity to reflect on what is important to you from the object of your desire. Also remember that whether you are looking to find, mend or maintain a loving relationship, you are half of that equation and until you love you, there will always be barriers blocking your way.

TAKEAWAY LESSON: If you are one half of a partnership, you both have equal responsibility to treat each other and yourself with the respect you deserve. Remember, we teach people how to treat us.

FAMILY MOON

Considering your Family Moon is a really good opportunity to think about how you interact with your kids if you have them, as well as your brothers, sisters, cousins, aunties, uncles and of course your parents. Parents. Can't live with 'em and can't exist without 'em. Put simply, setting goals when it comes to our creators is often a minefield; so tread carefully as the underlying issues that dictate family dynamics are often so deeply buried that you'd need an archaeologist on the level of Indiana Jones to venture into these ancient ruins. As a result, time spent with family can often be such a teeth-grinding affair that we leave their company exhausted, resentful and vowing that, 'Next Christmas, we are going abroad!' However, by setting some simple goals to improve the family unit, we can ensure that we share good experiences with these people rather than just DNA.

At this point, if you are thinking, 'Wasn't this supposed to be a book about food and fitness?', know that the relationships we have with the people in our lives have massive repercussions for how we treat ourselves. So, if every time you get off the phone to your sister you find yourself standing in front of the fridge reaching for a can of whipped cream, it could be that there is an underlying anxiety about the interaction that is driving you to literally swallow your feelings. Dealing with fractured relationships outside might be the catalyst to a healthier relationship inside.

The golden rule for setting family goals is to remember at all times that we are responsible for our own actions and, more important, we cannot control anyone else's view of us. It is a message that actually extends to all relationships and not just family ones. Simply willing another person to change their ways will never work. Instead, you have to take ownership of your part in that relationship, adapt your approach and be patient that eventually they will see that you are a different person. Of course, when it comes to our parents perhaps they will always see us as little kids and when you say, 'Mother, I have been reviewing our relationship dynamic and am committed to resolving our differences,' she probably hears, 'Look, Mummy, I just did a big poo-poo!'

Sometimes we don't help ourselves in this dynamic and even now whenever I visit my family home, I find myself regressing to a stroppy teenager with a quick temper and a habit of throwing out food orders from the couch. Maybe setting a goal to behave in a way that engenders respect rather than having a tantrum would help our parents see us as equals.

Even if, like me, you had a happy childhood and a great relationship with your family, there may be things you'd like to tweak, do more often or try to avoid. Setting conscious goals around the frequency and quality of family contact can have a massive impact. Think about your walk home from work. Could you set a goal that every day on this walk you are going to phone home and check in with the mother ship? Doing this every day will allow for relaxed small talk about nothing in particular rather than infrequent calls where bigger issues may need to be aired or built-up tension released.

Also, a large dollop of empathy is needed so we can reframe our parents not as supreme beings expected to be perfect but as humans who sometimes fuck up. And if you believe your parents messed up, then remember that for all their perceived failures, your parents for the most part did the best they could. If as a result of their actions you feel you have been wounded, let down, or lacking in life then perhaps now is the time to switch those negatives into positives.

In other words, instead of lamenting your parents' mistakes, think of the positive qualities that emerged from the embers of a fiery parent–child relationship. For example, instead of saying, 'My mum or dad did not spend enough time with me', and resenting them for it, reframe how you look at their neglect by declaring, 'My parents unwittingly gave me important life lessons about self-sufficiency and resilience.' Once you switch the words in your story, you'll see it can very quickly change for the better.

The real tragedy is that if parent–child issues are left unresolved it can often mean a lifetime of passive-aggressive jousting and when the parents pass away, their children are left even more resentful than before they died, robbed of an opportunity to set the record straight. Make the effort while you still can!

On the other hand, family goals might be more about kids than parents. After all, if you feel that your folks made mistakes raising you then you should be doubly mindful of how your behaviour will impact your children in the years to come. Additionally, setting some parenting goals with your partner is a great way to introduce them to the world of conscious goal-setting.

TAKEAWAY LESSON: We are responsible for our own actions and, more important, we cannot control anyone else's view of us.

FRIENDSHIP MOON

The way your Friendship Moon orbits Planet You can have a massive impact on how successfully you achieve your goals. It even determines the type of goals you might set in the first place – we care a lot about what our friends think and if they are quick to shun an idea, it can lead us to do the same too. This leads me on to the importance of making friends with people who elevate you (and who you can elevate in return) rather than associating with those who might hold you back, bring you down or unconsciously wound you.

After all, we all know a good friendship is based on trust, mutual support and positive experiences, yet when put under the microscope, not all of our friends behave in a friendly way. It is so easy to forget that unlike our family, we choose our friends, which means we can choose to break friendships as easily as we make them. This might seem controversial or even cold-hearted, yet if there are people in your life who don't make you happy then, just like Gwynnie and Chris, you owe it to yourself to consciously uncouple and move on.

The reason friends can affect us so much is because during an interaction with our BFFs we will instinctively mirror their behaviour, body language and even facial expressions as a way to bond and display unity. Yet this goes further than simple outward mirroring because we often mirror their emotions as well their behaviours, which ultimately we internalise and take away with us. It is a phenomenon called 'social contagion', so named because, like a virus, emotions literally spread from one person to another. This makes it vital to our psychological wellbeing to try to 'catch' uplifting emotions rather than get infected with negative ones.

If you are still not convinced, just picture your closest gal pals. Is there one in particular who regularly has news of a self-constructed dilemma or seemingly unjust conflict that is proof of her worthlessness and life's futility? What's more, despite her unhappiness, can you think of an occasion when she genuinely made an effort to change her circumstances or a time she showed gratitude for all the good things in her life? If the answer is 'yes' to the first question and 'no' to the second, you may need to stock up on garlic, get a vial of holy water and dial 0800-VAN-HELSING because you have undoubtedly fallen prey to an energy vampire, or Evie for short.

Evie is a friend in permanent crisis, a creature who (in my best David Attenborough voice) will gently coil around her prey before sinking her fangs into her victim's delicate skin, slowly yet ravenously draining its life blood. She won't take everything, just enough to leave her victim feeling lethargic, light-headed and looking for ways to solve her unresolvable issues.

The only way to avoid being feasted on is distance, both physical and emotional. This means minimising face-to-face contact, not indulging her needy texts and even unfollowing her on social media. It might seem harsh, yet Evie dines on turmoil and no matter how much you try to help, the chances are you won't get through. Worse still, by being complicit in her misery addiction you'll be unwittingly reinforcing her cycle of negative behaviour.

It can prove difficult as by the time you get into your forties and beyond, many of your friends may be lifelong acquaintances, so it can be hard to imagine an escape from such history. If you're in this position, it's important to remember that a shared past does not have to dictate a shared future, which is especially pertinent if you want to make some big life changes.

The good news is that happiness is just as contagious as negativity, so catch a dose and also make an effort to spread as much as you can. Set some goals that involve replacing energy sappers with energy zappers and join clubs and classes that will attract like-minded people interested in looking forward rather than backwards.

If you already have great friends who lift you up, then set goals to see them more often or change up the things you do together. Better still, involve them in your goal-setting as it is easier to buddy up and also adds a layer of accountability (more on that later).

TAKEAWAY LESSON: Just because you have shared memories and events with someone, that does not mean you owe them your energy for life. Replace sappers with zappers.

BODY MOON

It's OK to want to change the way we look, so shed the shame from setting Body Moon goals right now. After all, achieving body goals can work wonders for our self-esteem and personal confidence levels and I bet even the most enlightened Buddhist monk meditating in a Tibetan monastery in the Himalayan mountains still looks at their reflection from time to time and asks, 'Does my bum look big in this?' We just need to be careful that the goal doesn't become a fixation and that the achievement of this goal does not take over our lives because we'll miss out on so much as a result.

For all its complexities, your brain will basically push you towards pleasure and away from pain. However, if we focus too much on running away from pain, then no matter how close to pleasure we get, we'll always be looking backwards in fear that the pain will return. For example, if your 'pain' is your love handles, bingo wings or muffin top and you are always creating goals designed to minimise that pain, then every time you think about a trip to the gym or a run around the block you'll be glued to that narrative.

Then, even when you achieve that particular body goal, you'll still be stuck on the same record and worried about the consequences of that pain (in this case, fat) potentially returning. Eventually, you'll be so terrified, your whole life will revolve around avoiding that pain regardless of the consequences. I've been there and you know what? It sucks.

I switched it by setting positive body goals based on improving and maintaining my overall health, rather than pushing myself to alleviate the 'pain' which in my case was belly flab, bigger thighs and being larger than a size 8. I realised that healthy bodies look like healthy bodies and that I couldn't keep focusing on the 'physical flaws' I'd got so worked up about over the years. I concentrated on a balanced diet, moderate levels of exercise, less stress and more sleep. Most of all, I worked out that if we live in a world geared around the escape from pain, then no matter how good life gets, we'll always be living in fear.

In practical terms, I began to make this switch by treating my Body Moon goals in terms of numbers (quantitative) rather what I saw in the mirror (qualitative). So instead of judging my success by my reflection, I thought of other health measures I could work towards, such as my cholesterol levels, VO2 max test (the maximum amount of oxygen you can use during exercise) or the number of seconds I could hold a plank. I also set body goals around the way I moved, rather than how I looked, which led me to include things like Pilates so that I could address imbalances that were impairing my mobility. Most of all, I listened to my body and set balanced goals to include rest days, stretch days and days when my body goals could take a back seat guilt-free.

Now a word of warning ... whatever you do, don't use a weighing scales as part of your body goals! While your weight is indeed a quantitative measure, it does not accurately reflect a person's health. For example, Linford Christie is a 100m Olympic sprinter, while Phil 'The Power' Taylor is an international darts player. Say that both of them have identical numbers when they stand on the weighing scales – I know which one I'd choose to run up ten flights of stairs and rescue me from a burning building!

Muscle weighs more than fat, so that fact alone should be enough of an indication that losing weight is not always great. Your weight can fluctuate depending on the time of the day or even your 'time of the month', so focusing too closely on interpreting these numbers will drive you crazy. If you want to lose weight I would recommend opting to test your cholesterol level because measurements such as this will only go down if you improve your overall lifestyle for a sustained period in a healthy way. It has the added bonus of accountability (we'll get to that in a bit) because having to take the blood test means going to your GP. Furthermore, you'll need to discuss the results with your doctor and then have a follow-up consultation in six months, which will give you a definite target to aim for.

TAKEAWAY LESSON: Where body image is concerned, set positive goals based on a move towards a better life rather than negative ones based on escaping pain.

As Cindy Lauper once said, 'When the working day is done, oh girls, they wanna have fun.' So wise. So true. Rest and play might not seem like something we need to set active goals for, but if we neglect to unplug, switch off or tune out, our mental and physical health can take a sudden nose dive. That's why our Fun Moon is such an important one.

Yet as kick-ass 21st-century women we often get down about our down time and feel that leisure time is wasted time. That is just not the case, so say it with me, ladies, 'down time is divine time', so heavenly in fact that it even says in the Bible, 'There is a time to toil and a time to chill the fuck out!' or something to that effect.

There should be things we all do in our daily lives that we do purely for the joy of it. Not because they lead somewhere or because they tick a box, but because we all need to allow our inner child to come out to play from time to time. The difficulty arises from the fact that as adults, there is always something to do on the to-do list, so the best way to ensure playtime exists is to organise it in advance.

Additionally, you could set a Fun Moon goal to rekindle a love for a long-lost hobby or sport you played as a child but then gave up as a teenager when you switched after-school tennis lessons for after-school French lessons behind the bike sheds. Hobbies are so useful because they centre your breathing and absorb your entire focus, allowing the woes of the outside world to take a back seat. And if that sounds like a textbook definition of meditation, that's because it is. After all, meditation doesn't have to be about crossed legs, incense and a bearded guru – it can just as easily involve crossed knitting needles, a ball of wool and your bearded gran. And all those years you thought she was knitting oversized sweaters just for you, she was ascending to a higher plane of consciousness, quietly observing her own paradigm! Far out, Gran.

Above all, regardless of whether you are setting goals to have structured fun or want to sneak into an afternoon screening of *Fifty Shades of Grey* once in a while, don't feel guilty for taking the time to play, because experiencing anxiety around relaxing defeats the purpose.

Better still, set some new experiential leisure goals, thereby creating new memories – from simple trips to the theatre to finally taking that dream holiday you've been talking about for years and never got around to. Doing so could also have a positive effect on your love life, friendships and family relationships as you move along the path from box sets to bucket lists and beyond. The important thing to remember is that not all goals need to feel like work. Planning fun will also prevent weekends slipping by or paid holidays being squandered in a panic of aggressive vegging out on the couch (while still most likely checking work emails).

TAKEAWAY LESSON: Setting goals for the fun area of our lives is just as important as other, more worthy-sounding goals, because that is the area we tend to neglect.

MIND MOON

Last but by no means least, the Mind Moon refers to everything that is going on between your ears – and I don't mean your sassy new hairdo. Whether it is breaking a bad habit, learning something new, like an instrument, language or skill, or simply learning to listen to what's going on inside your thoughts, the Mind Moon is a crucial part of goal-setting because your inner narrative is where all your personal goals are forged and hopefully achieved.

The Mind Moon is also a perfect example of how setting a goal in one orbit can help you to achieve your goals in other orbits without you even having to try. Let's say you choose the Mind Moon goal to go sober for six months. The consequences of this commitment will immediately ripple out into every aspect of your lifestyle because, first, alcohol costs money. Therefore, the Money Moon goal you set to ensure there was an extra five thousand quid in your savings account by your birthday looks a lot more doable when you realise that the bucks you spent on booze will now stay in your account. It all adds up – from the two bottles of red during the week, to the hundreds you spend on Friday night cocktails, as well as a few glasses of Pimm's and lemonade with Sunday lunch. When totalled, you suddenly realise that in the space of just half a year, by switching your cocktails to mocktails you will be saving over four grand!

Meanwhile, your professional life is on the up because without the interrupted sleep and constant hangovers, you are more productive at work. The increased sharpness and productivity mean that all of a sudden the Money Moon goal to get promoted is also looking more realistic. What's more, if the big promotion doesn't come your way, you now have the confidence to revisit your CV and start looking for a job that will give you greater satisfaction.

Alternatively, we could investigate how the chances of succeeding at your Love Moon goals have suddenly been boosted by your decision to quit the shandy. Let's say instead of leaving the money you save in the bank, you decide to use the extra cash to fund your goal to spend quality time with your partner by visiting one new European city every month. Now you'll be making new memories, shaking up a routine and exploring the world together.

It might not all be roses because without the boozy nights, you might find the relationship has a void that can't be filled by sober fun, so be warned. Hopefully, he/she comes along for the ride and is open to the idea of self-empowerment, but there are no guarantees and ultimately you might find that this is not the person to sail off into the sunset with.

The same goes for your Friendship Moon. When I set my goal to leave the hangovers in the past, I found some friends weren't ready to accept that and I found myself at the wrong end of more than the odd social snubbing. That's OK because I made new friends who share my core values and who I can get into all sorts of adventures with, that years ago I would have simply dismissed.

Quitting the booze will also have your Body Moon rejoicing, because you will not be indulging in those Friday night Chinese takeaways with their thousands of empty calories. Plus, now you've reclaimed your Saturday mornings, which means more time and energy to go and get some exercise, further helping you to achieve your body goals.

Then think about your Family Moon, which gets more attention because without the late rising and banging headache, you can spend more time with your kids, FaceTime your folks and grab some brunch with your sister.

Then during Sunday lunch at the in-laws, you notice you're more patient and even-tempered and furthermore you are able to spot triggers and not rise to anger when old scabs are picked at.

TAKEAWAY LESSON: As you can see, your life is interconnected and making positive decisions in one area of your life will have a ripple effect and positive ramifications for all aspects of your life.

ASSESS, ACCURACY AND ACCOUNTABILITY

And so we move on to the A in GOALS, or should I say three As, because this next phase involves a few different steps, where you'll review and refine your 28 goals, elevating them from vague desires to accurate and accountable goals. The aim of this is to get you to where you want to go as well as giving you the confidence, patience and serenity to forget the final destination altogether and just enjoy the journey.

ASSESS

First, you need to assess and understand what is important to you at this moment of your life in a non-critical and judgement-free way. This exercise is simple and you have already done most of the work for this when you wrote out your 28 goals and gave each one a number. These numbers can be stacked to make a bar graph with the seven lunar orbits along the bottom and the goals stacked one on top of the other. See the example on page 151.

By the end of the process, you might be surprised to see that one orbit is particularly dominant, or notice areas of your life that are under-serviced. For example, the graph on page 151 is from a friend of mine, who appears to be (from the distribution of her goals) something of a workaholic. As you can see, the goals are heavily skewed towards perceived productivity, financial gain and body-oriented goals with almost no emphasis on fun, love, friendship or family. Just completing this exercise was really helpful for her, as it got her to realise that she needed to reassess her priorities.

Remember, there are no judgements here, so please do not get downhearted if you end up with 28 goals in one category and nothing in any of the others. Instead, use it as an opportunity to address any imbalances by going back to your list and adding a few goals in the areas that are currently being neglected.

Once you have balanced your graph a little, you need to pick **ONE GOAL FROM EACH ORBIT** to focus on. That isn't to say that all the others will be disregarded for all eternity, simply that even if you have a completely balanced graph, it would be asking a lot to set 28 goals all on the same day.

MONEY MOON	LOVE MOON	FAMILY MOON	FRIENDSHIP MOON	BODY MOON	FUN MOON	MIND MOON
				28		
26				25		
20				21		
14				19		
13				15		
10				9		
7			27	8		23
2	22	24	17	5		18
1	11	12	3	4	16	6

How you choose this is up to you, just be mindful not to disregard goals you 'don't have time for' – the biggest trap to fall into is to change your goals to fit into your lifestyle rather than changing your lifestyle to make room for your new goals. After all, this is a process that involves growth and progressing rather than plateauing. Strap on your boots and take a big step out of your comfort zone.

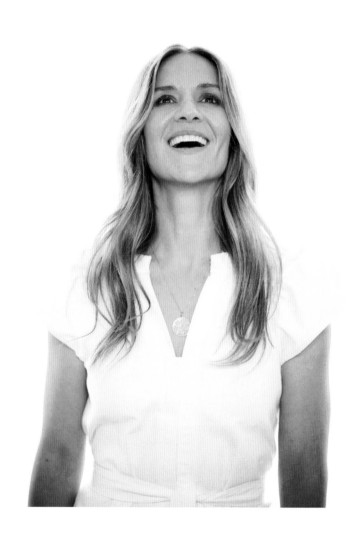

Once you have chosen one goal from each orbit most worthy of your time and energy, (never forget that these are *your* goals, no one else's) it is time to get accurate and hone them from being vague desires into precise blueprints for success.

ACCURACY

Look at what you have written. You will notice that they all have one thing in common: they all come under the banner, 'I am here, and I want to get there.' It is a very simple desire. However, the simplicity of the desire can also be its downfall, because while it gives us a start point and an end point, it fails to give us a plan of how to get there, how long it will take to get there and why we are even setting that goal in the first place. For example, you don't just get into a taxi and say 'drive'. Instead, you give the taxi driver a specific address, an exact postcode for his GPS and if time is an issue, let him know you need to arrive by a certain time. Therefore, it is not enough to just say, 'I want more money', you must be more specific about how much money you want, how quickly you want it and, most important, how the hell you are going to get it! Is it through saving more or spending less? Will you be earning a larger wage or quitting your job and setting up a business?

This is also where NLP comes in handy (see page 84) because you'll need to review the language used in each goal and ensure you are using the right words, at the right time and in the right way. This might involve reframing the desire so that it is driving towards a positive goal rather than a negative one. For example, in the past you might have set the goal to 'lose weight', which not only is a negative target, it doesn't offer any indication of *why* you want to lose it and *how* you intend losing it. Is it through switching your diet? Is it through increasing your exercise? Is it through switching your mealtimes? Is it through switching your portion sizes? Or is it all of the above? More important, rather than fixating on the weight loss, wouldn't it be better to set a positive goal and allow the weight loss to be a beneficial side effect?

So instead of focusing on weight loss, set a goal based on improving fitness. Thus the positive and accurate version of 'I want to lose weight', would instead sound something like this, 'For the next 14 days, I will set my alarm 30 minutes earlier than usual and use that time to get out of bed and do a mini exercise circuit.' Not a single mention of weight loss or dropping a dress size and yet if you incorporate this small circuit into your daily life, you'll soon notice results.

Here are a few more examples of vague goals that can be rewritten to offer more clarity on what the goal is and also how to achieve it:

ORIGINAL GOAL: 'I want to drink more water.'

ORIGINAL GOAL: 'I want to be calmer.'

REVIEW: 'How much water is "more" and when will I drink this throughout the day?'

REVIEW: 'How do I define "calm" and what makes me calm?'

ACCURATE GOAL: 'For seven days before I go to sleep, I will place a 1 litre bottle of water beside my bed. When I wake up and before I get out of bed, I will sip this until it is finished.'

ACCURATE GOAL: 'For the next seven days, every night at 9 p.m. I will turn off the TV/laptop/iPhone and spend 10 minutes breathing deeply.'

Look back at how these goals have changed and marvel at the difference. All of a sudden they have gone from vague statements to accurate blueprints for success that tick all the boxes!

✔ Quantitative? CHECK!

✔ Accurate? CHECK!

✔ A realistic time frame? CHECK!

✔ A goal that reframes the narrative? CHECK!

That's more checks than a bistro in Prague! One thing these don't have is accountability, which although is not vital, is a useful tool in following a plan through.

ACCOUNTABILITY

Unplanned promises made on a whim are as easy to break as they are to make. So being held accountable is crucial for the discipline to continue. The easiest way to find accountability is to select a friend, loved one or even a professional to whom you declare your intention and who will then act as a walking, talking conscience. It might even inspire them to join in and then you can benefit from the bonus of having a companion to inspire you when you feel like giving in.

A classic example of accountability for a goal is to sign up for a planned event such as a marathon. Each year, thousands of first-timers sign up months in advance and then work diligently towards achieving this goal. They might be sponsored, adding further responsibility, and even if they are doing it purely to participate, the idea of a definite goal, on a specific date and with the eyes of the world watching can be a very powerful motivator. Now, you might feel that a marathon is a step, or 60,000 steps to be precise, too far and want to start with a 5km run or even walk.

Of course there is not the equivalent of a marathon for every aspect of your life, so adding accountability to other goals can take a little more invention. For example, there are a few different tactics you could employ to help you on your quest for a digital detox. First, you can use your phone by changing the settings to minimise your screen time. You might find this is so easy to circumvent that the slight nuisance is not enough to deter you. Next you might try deleting the relevant app from your smartphone altogether, only to find that you are still finding ways to get online and check your feed. Perhaps it is time for something more drastic and for this you'll need the help of a friend you trust ... and by trust I mean *really* trust because you'll need to give them your login details so they can change your password, effectively shutting you out of your account for an agreed length of time, say four weeks. That means you won't be able to like, comment or post without going to them for permission to login. You have heard of Dry January and Sober October, well how about DigiDetox December or NoSocial September? The key is that by relinquishing control and handing a trusted friend the keys, you no longer have to fight the unconscious urge, which could give you just enough breathing space to kick the habit for good.

You might even inspire your friend to do the same and give you the password to her social media account, meaning that you'll be encouraging each other to stay the course.

Even if you don't find a pal or professional to hold you accountable, it is important that you keep the promises you make to yourself. Something as simple as writing down your daily progress in the form of a journal can help you do this. Diarising your thoughts is also a great way to start a dialogue with yourself in a way that allows you to be completely honest about what you are thinking, how that makes you feel and why you're on that path. The time you spend writing your journal will also be therapeutic as you clear your mind of the day's distractions and take a little time to digest.

ASSESS AGAIN

Now that you have one accurate goal from each orbit, assign a day of the week on which to check in with that goal and perform a mini audit. So, for example, on Monday you might take a moment to assess your Family Moon goal, on Tuesday perhaps you want to analyse your Fun Moon goal, Wednesday your Body Moon goal and so on. You might find after an initial audit that the goal you set was both unrealistic and too difficult or, by contrast, unchallenging and too easy. That's OK, tweak as you go – it's all a part of the process, designed to incorporate the goals into your lifestyle.

LIFESTYLE

You might think fitting all these goals into your day-to-day would be too much, so make it as easy as possible for yourself by breaking down your goals into their simplest parts. That way you won't feel overwhelmed before you have even had a chance to begin.

For example, say you set a goal to improve your posture. Where to even begin? Your head might start spinning while you consider whether to opt for trips to the chiropractor, go online to download volumes of reading about biomechanics, or sign up to a Pilates class. All of these solutions would work but incorporating them into a productive lifestyle will take time, energy, money and such a serious balancing act that you might conclude it's just not worth the effort. Instead, consider your current lifestyle and how you could mould it around this new goal.

One suggestion could be to focus on standing up straight each time you brush your teeth. Easy as that! That would equate to two minutes every morning and another two minutes every evening when you are consciously focusing on how you are standing with your feet shoulder-width apart, hips in neutral, core engaged and breathing from your stomach. Do that and you will have gifted yourself with four minutes a day of Pilates without very little effort. That translates to almost 30 minutes a week! All for free and during a time when you would otherwise have been mindlessly brushing with one hand and scrolling through *The Guardian* online with the other.

In time, this 'mindful' standing could extend to other seemingly mundane moments in your life such as waiting at the bus stop or queuing at the supermarket or coffee shop. Do this every day and before long, you will be naturally standing in a more upright and engaged way, which will lead to a better posture, deeper breathing patterns and improved muscle tone and blood flow. All without you breaking a sweat or changing your schedule to accommodate your new aim!

An added bonus of making these little habits a part of your everyday routine is that if you do them deliberately enough times they get absorbed into the fabric of your personality. For instance, I no longer think about getting my five-a-day because at some point in the past this conscious daily effort became an unconscious, instinctive habit that happens without a second thought.

Remember, if your knee-jerk reaction is 'I don't have time' or 'This goal does not fit into my life,' then *make* time, lady! I will add that it is important to have realistic goals. This is your long game, and by long game I don't mean, 'Next weekend when I go to Moira's hen do in Marbella I want to look like Kate Moss,' I mean the looooong game; being whole, complete and happy for life.

It's also important to be realistic about your goals – setting unrealistic goals will needlessly reduce your chances of success from the get-go. For example, you've just had a baby and you want to shift the baby weight ASAP – you can't wait to get your pre-baby bod back. Well, stop, look in the mirror and own the following two truths before you do anything:

❶ Nothing is going to happen in the first few weeks of your newborn's life, because you simply won't have the time to exercise.

❷ You will most likely be exhausted from sleepless nights and super-emotional from a cocktail of hormones surging through your body, so you will need all your energy just to get through the days.

So what is realistic? Could it be setting out some times when you can walk outdoors with your baby? Or perhaps set a schedule where you can do some light exercises in the living room as baby sleeps? You have to decide what works for you during this time of upheaval and not put too much pressure on yourself.

Ultimately, the aim of conscious goal-setting is not to improve your life but to improve your *lifestyle*. This means incorporating small changes on a regular basis into your daily/weekly routine, all the time keeping in mind that life is not something any of us can have 100 per cent control over and shit, as they say, happens.

SMALL STEPS

Start slowly with small steps and graduate at your own pace. Remember, these are your goals and once you incorporate them into your lifestyle, remain patient – you can always re-evaluate them as you go. That is not giving you carte blanche to give up the first time the going gets tough, just a reminder that any worthwhile changes you make in your life, especially when it comes to retraining behaviour patterns, will not happen overnight and if you expect too much too soon you'll get disheartened and throw in the towel. The trick is to take it one day at a time and not focus on the actual goal at all. That way you avoid getting fixated on the final destination and missing out on the journey.

The journey towards the goal is extremely important, because that is your day-to-day experience of life! The last thing you want to do is to wish away the hours, days, months and years, desperately waiting for the day you achieve your goals. For example, when I first started writing this book I couldn't imagine how I was ever going to hit my word count. Those first couple of weeks were probably the cleanest my kitchen has ever been as I found every excuse under the sun to avoid tackling such a momentous undertaking. Then I remembered that a book is made up of chapters, which are made up of pages, and paragraphs and sentences and words and letters, so all I had to do was write the first line. As it happened, I deleted that line about two minutes later, but I had taken the first step and that was all I could hope for in that moment. In time, those first words I put on the page were joined by others and after days, weeks and months, that first line swelled into something I never believed possible.

The same is true of all our goals: you need to break down how best to achieve a goal into its simplest parts (in my case, words) and to deal with just the bit that is right in front of you. If you have ever seen an ant on a nature programme, you'll see where I'm coming from.

Another part of the small-steps mentality is that you can reward yourself! You deserve tangible treats along the way. I'm talking gold stars for goal stars, ladies! Get yourself a calendar and a bag of gold stars and every day you successfully complete a goal-related activity, give yourself a shiny star sticker. You remember that feeling when you got them as a kid? It was amazing to know that you had earned the shiny badge of honour and just that feeling was enough.

It might seem silly at first but I guarantee that in all of us there is a little child who loves the recognition, so give in to that feeling and enjoy the moment. Also, gold stars can be traded for anything you like, from trips to the movies, to that cardi you spotted at H&M, to booking tickets to go to that band you always wanted to see.

A word of warning, though: making your rewards food-related is a bad idea. It promotes food as something that is withheld or to be indulged in, depending on your perceived success and general behaviour. Doing this can create all sorts of unconscious connections that spill over and cause distress without you even knowing it. It's called 'behavioural conditioning', made famous by a Russian called Ivan Pavlov with the help of his bitch, a bell and a biscuit ... and I don't mean his girlfriend! (By all accounts Ivan was a gentleman and respected all the ladies in his life.) Pavlov conducted a behavioural conditioning experiment where he rang a bell every time he fed his canine assistant a biscuit. Naturally the dog salivated because she was excited for the treat and the next day, Pavlov rang the bell again and offered another biscuit. Over the next few days every time he offered her the tasty treat he rang the bell and eventually just the sound of the bell would make her salivate even when no biscuit was present. The conclusion was that Pavlov's dog had learned to associate the bell with the biscuit and the truth is that, although you ain't no bitch, sister, you are likely to associate certain stimuli with certain behaviours and emotions, so it is really important not to create triggers that work against you in the long run.

NLP alert ...this is another reason why I stopped using the phrase 'cheat day' because cheating implies something underhanded, dishonest or forbidden and associating those feelings with food made me feel guilty in the aftermath. Once I had my Switch moment, I realised that when it comes to the way I want to think about my meal choices, the last thing I should want to do is delight in dishonesty. That creates the sort of confused internal dialogue Mrs Zippy used to thrive on. She revelled in the reward and then chastised me for being a morally bankrupt weakling.

Now you have everything you need to set goals successfully. With a little bit of time, thought and honesty you will be setting and achieving goals in no time. So get your pen and paper make that Switch. Here's a recap:

1   Splurge out 28 goals; number them as you go (don't think about it too hard).

2   Organise the goals into a lunar orbits bar graph (see page 151) with the headings: Money, Love, Family, Friendship, Body, Fun and Mind Moons.

3   Use the lunar orbits along the bottom and begin to stack the goals (using the number of the goal instead of writing out the whole goal.

4   Use the graph as a visual indicator to review how your goals are balanced across the different aspects of your life. In other words, are you fixating on one and neglecting others?

5   Now pick ONE goal from each category and make these your seven primary goals.

6   Look at each of these seven goals and make sure they are accurate blueprints rather than vague desires.

7   Make sure you can be held accountable for them.

8   Consider and understand how you can incorporate these into your daily lifestyle or how your daily life needs to change to achieve your goals. Remember; push yourself to step out of your comfort zone.

9   Take small steps and remember to reward yourself as you go.

10 Check in frequently to review and revise your goals without attaching judgement, guilt or shame. This is called 'auditing'. You have seven goals and seven days in the week, so audit one of your goals every day.

MONEY MOON	LOVE MOON	FAMILY MOON	FRIENDSHIP MOON	BODY MOON	FUN MOON	MIND MOON

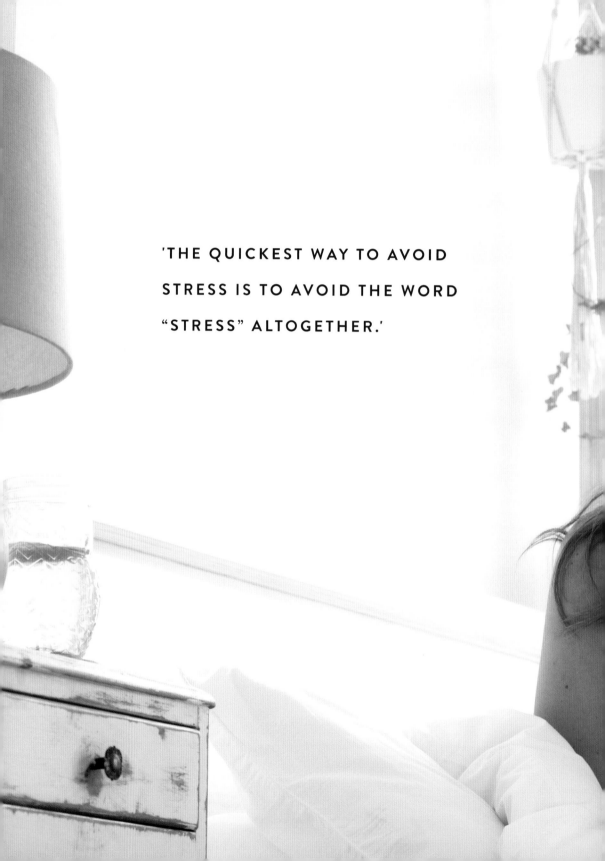

'THE QUICKEST WAY TO AVOID
STRESS IS TO AVOID THE WORD
"STRESS" ALTOGETHER.'

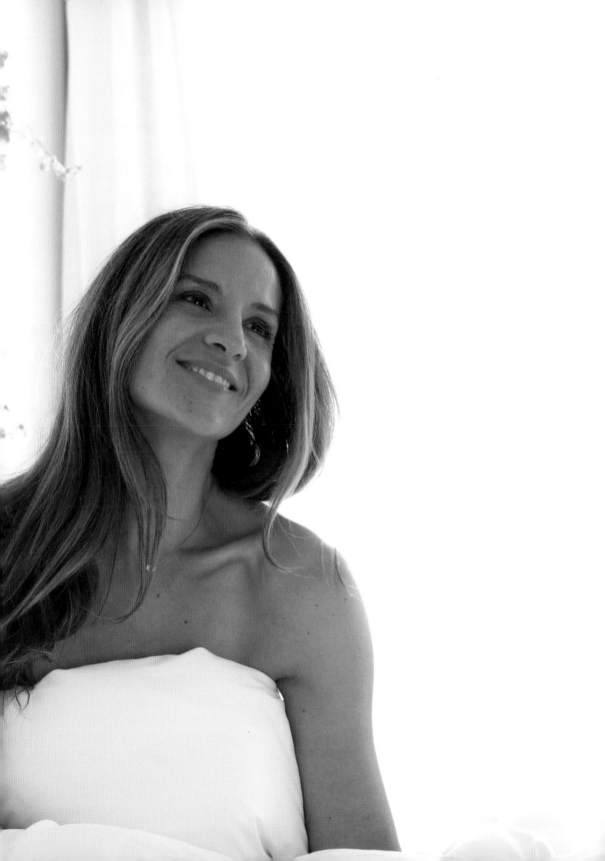

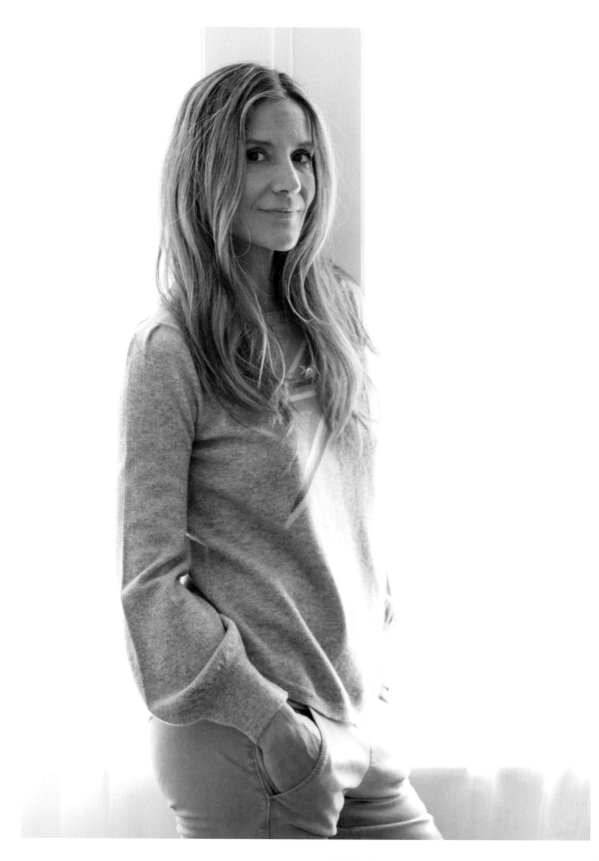

ZEN:

THE ART OF BEING

PEACEFUL AND RELAXED

$\longleftrightarrow$

NOW IT'S TIME to learn the benefits of truly winding down and being at peace with yourself and the world. You will find that if you swerve stress, avoid anxiety, master mindfulness and sleep soundly, your work day and your 'me time' will thrive and you will be on your way to a healthier, happier you in no time.

LET'S TALK ABOUT STRESS, BABY

—

Stress is not a medically defined condition. It is instead a side-effect of the body's fight or flight response and it is how we interpret the experience that matters. You might be surprised to hear that stress can be good – in small doses this physical reaction can help you to focus, excel and generally get shit done. There was a time when this response was a life-or-death survival tool but in modern life, there are thankfully very few occasions when we genuinely need this reaction. The problem occurs when we use the word 'stress' for simple daily trip-ups that are not consistent with the situation. Do this too often and it can really damage your mind as well as your body.

The long-term physical effects of unchecked stress include suppressed immunity, burnouts, breakdowns and hormonal imbalances, also known as adrenal fatigue. This string of woes becomes all the more upsetting when you consider that a lot of the stress we experience is self-inflicted.

For example, if you have a deadline at work it may cause you to feel 'stressed'. But in reality the emotion you are experiencing is only your mind's reminder that this work matters, so it is time to put away your toys and get down to it. Getting wound up about it will not push the deadline or get the work done but if we keep telling ourselves how 'stressed' we are about it, two things will happen:

❶   It will trigger a learned response that the situation is worthy of panic.

❷   It will actually impair our ability to succeed, creating a feedback loop that is hard to escape from.

So how do we avoid this whirlpool of woe?

COPING STRATEGIES FOR WHEN STRESS WELLS UP

There are a number of coping strategies you can employ to help you break the cycle and forge ahead in a state of Zen.

PULL THE TRIGGER WORD

The quickest way to avoid 'stress' is to avoid the word 'stress' altogether. Just stating expressions such as, 'I'm stressed', 'You're stressing me out' or 'This is stressful' are enough to conjure up feelings of anxiety and a mild sense of panic.

As I explained in Neuro-Linguistic Programming (see page 84), instead of saying, 'I feel stressed', switch it out for something fun that makes you smile. 'I feel funky, maybe I'll have little dance to this funky feeling while I figure it out.'

Applying this technique to the deadline example, you will suddenly realise that if it is not met, you will not spontaneously combust and rather than get worked up, you will smile to yourself and get down to work.

A useful technique when your thoughts are feeling out of control is the 'salty water' visualisation. For this, imagine that your mind is a crystal-clear glass of water and life stresses are grains of salt. Add a little, and the grains of salt will dissolve effortlessly. However, if you dump in a spoonful all at once and stir it up, the result is a whirlpool of cloudy water, spinning uncontrollably. The solution is to stop, visualise yourself taking the metaphorical spoon out the glass and with each breath, picture the whirlpool getting slower until it eventually disappears. Once you have mindfully made the whirlpool vanish, continue to breathe deeply and imagine the salt settling to the bottom of the glass. Eventually, the water returns to crystal clarity, allowing you to see clearly once more.

This is a very powerful visualisation, so the next time life dumps a spoonful of salty stress into your glass and your mind feels like a spinning vortex, picture it slowing, stopping and the water returning to clarity. This cannot be rushed. Remember, 'Stirring it up will not your problems solve, instead you just need to slow down and let it dissolve.'

TO BREATHE OR NOT TO BREATHE?
(THAT'S NOT EVEN A QUESTION)

Without breath there is no life. How long can you hold your breath? For me, it's about 45 seconds. When you are feeling 'funky', you'll notice the first thing to suffer is your breathing pattern. Breathing gets shorter and shallower and perhaps you experience a pain in your chest. The physical reaction can lead to a psychological one as your brain has literally less oxygen to think. The quickest way to get back on an even keel is with deep, mindful breathing.

This allows the heart to slow and can lower blood pressure, increase your energy levels, improve your blood flow, stimulate the lymphatic system and even improve digestion. So any time you feel funky, stop, close your eyes, take deep breaths through your belly, and move on.

MEDITATE ON THAT

Experts believe that we have an average of 70,000 thoughts a day – that's an average of 2,900 an hour, which is 48 thoughts a minute ... A MINUTE! That's a lot of thoughts to process and many of them can be negative, so you can see why taking a moment to learn how to meditate – to stop thinking of anything at all, for a brief moment, can eventually bring your chatty mind to a standstill and give her a break from the mind gossip.

The simplest way to meditate is to sit quietly and focus on your breathing. If thoughts come rushing in, imagine them as weeds, and just pluck them out and discard them, then simply return to your breath. I know how hard it can be, because often when we sit in silence, we start to think of so many things. You're calm and focused and a plane goes overhead: 'Hmm, I wonder where that plane is going? I wish I were on a plane. Gosh, I can't wait for my holiday. I am not sure if I should be going with Greg, though. AGH. STOP. MEDITATE ... OK, I've got this!'

Have you ever noticed that some mundane daily tasks make you feel calm? Some people say washing up or hoovering has that effect on them. And the reason is because they are solely focused on the act, and do not let any other thoughts muddy the clean water of their thoughts. Absolutely every single one of us has the ability to meditate, and it's free! According to those who meditate daily, lives can be transformed and happiness happens as a by-product – with very little effort. I say Ommmm to that!

FUTURE YOU

When your mind starts spinning and you are feeling anxious, imagine a 'future you'. She is still you, just not the 'you' of the present. Instead, she is the 'you' of tomorrow, next week, next month, next year. 'Future you' will deal with everything in the future, not to be confused with 'present you', who is busy doing things in front of her and frankly has a lot to be getting on with. So I let 'Future Amanda' deal with future scenarios.

TAMING THE EGO

We are each the hero of our own story, and therefore we always assume we are right, even when we know we are wrong. If you find it too easy to get defensive and lash out, that's your ego playing up. The best way to deal with the ego is when you get irate, aggressive or argumentative, close your eyes, take a breath and recognise the trigger that's making you have the reaction (it might be your mother in law, it may be someone in a car in traffic, it may be someone accusing you of stealing their bench at the gym). Now, put a 'space' between you and the 'trigger'. That space could be an imaginary light, hand or wall. Now, tell your ego it's OK and that there is a physical object holding you back. And now for the hard part: apologise. Apologise either for your actions, or apologise for the other person's perception of your actions, and move on. This pause and acknowledgment is a huge step towards taming the ego and becoming happier, and saying sorry is one of the most liberating feelings you will ever experience.

THE FAST-FORWARD BUTTON

Sometimes a bad mood can stick around long after the initial grievance has passed. You can spend minutes, hours or days annoyed about a scenario and it affects every fibre of your being. Of course, eventually, the grump goes away, yet how long it lasted was entirely within your control even if it didn't feel like it in the moment. A great technique to help you to get from pissed off to peaceful more quickly, is the fast-forward button technique.

It works by imagining yourself sitting in a cinema and watching the current situation play out as though you are viewing a movie of your life. Although right now it might feel like you're in a horror flick, keep watching long enough and you'll soon be witnessing a comedy. With that in mind, you have two choices; either keep enduring the misery or to simply grab the remote and press the fast-forward button, skipping all the sadness in the process. Remember, you are the director of your life, so go get that Oscar, baby!

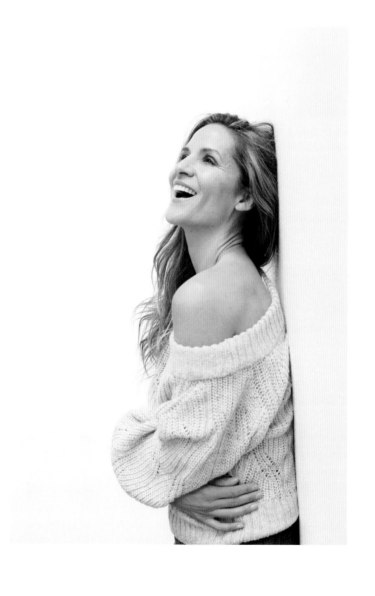

FINDING LONG-TERM ZEN

—

SWITCHING OFF SOCIAL MEDIA

Roll up, roll up. The School of Social Media is in session! Imagine a school with a totally toxic environment, where bullying is acceptable. A school where everything you say or believe in is up for scrutiny. At the end of each day an assembly is held where you stand under a spotlight and take criticism for how you looked, worked out, acted, what you did and said that day; basically how you live your life.

Each day the loudspeaker in the assembly would be taken over by the mean girls spewing and spitting fire about how great their lives are and how yours isn't, how ripped their abs are, and yours aren't, how happy their relationships are, and yours is not.

You absolutely hate this school and it makes you sad every morning you wake up and realise you have to go and be a part of it. You desperately want to leave the school, in fact you have tried to run away a few times and delete its address from your phone, but for some reason, you keep going back because you think that if you are not a part of it, you might be perceived as an outsider, a freak, someone who has no friends and no life.

Now, imagine it was you who applied to this school in the first place. It was you who sought it out, put your name down, gave your information, your photo albums, and it is you who updates it every day with your thoughts, your food preferences, your love life and sometimes your children's lives, even though you knew that sometimes the mean girls would scrutinise them.

And not just that, you stand by, you listen, you watch, and sometimes without even knowing it, you join in and become a part of the mean girl gang. Sometimes, other girls and boys, and often strangers, will tell you how much they love you. This makes you happy because the only thing you really want from this school is to be accepted, popular and loved. In fact just 'liked' will do – as many likes as possible.

If you haven't guessed by now, this school is an analogy for social media and it's often the worst kind of school, group, gang or community to be a part of. Yet we wake up every morning, put on our proverbial knee socks and line up back at the door again.

I myself am on social media; it is an integral part of my job, and so I completely understand the need to be involved, visible or at least connected. However, what is not healthy is engaging with it constantly, checking your phone, sharing untruthful, unrealistic, filtered posts. Stop comparing your life with others. Why try to fit in when you were born to stand out? Try spending less time on social media and caring less what anyone thinks of your photos and videos. You will find the path to Zen much more quickly.

SLEEP

Going to bed with too many thoughts can destroy a good night's sleep, and a bad night's sleep will ruin your day. You will be tired, run down, grumpy and reaching for those SADs (see page 49) just to get you through the day. It's also important not to watch TV in bed, and without a doubt, leave your phone in another room. Your phone, social media, emails, phone calls have absolutely no place in your sleep sanctuary. Seeing an email about work will spark your brain into productivity mode, and watching a video on social media will make you spiral into a plethora of thought patterns; the last thing you need before drifting off into a fluffy cloud nirvana. To convince you further, all of these devices emit blue light, which increases the risk of eyesight degeneration. Blue light also supresses melatonin, a hormone made by your brain that helps to control your daily sleep–wake cycles. This hero hormone is not only important for healthy sleep patterns, it is also anti-ageing, anti-inflammatory, and has antioxidant effects.

TIME OUT

In the western world we have become accustomed to living to work rather than working to live. Our work ethos has become obsessive and even when we try to pull back we are still constantly reachable via email, text or WhatsApp. As a consequence, we often find it hard to disconnect from work issues and work-related anxieties.

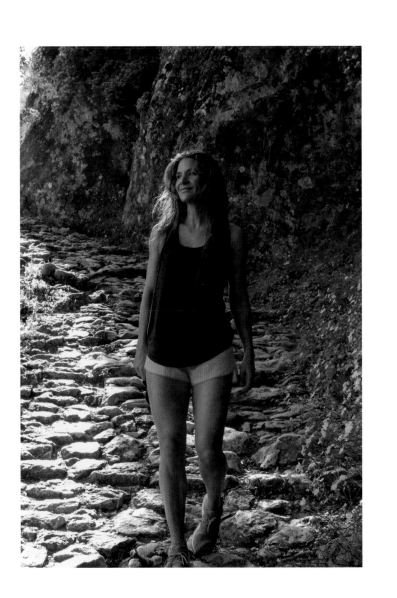

Each day many of us, like a flock of loyal sheep, set off on trains, trams or buses or sit in bumper-to-bumper traffic. On the journey, we often get squashed by the crowds as if we were penguins huddled together on the coldest day in the Antarctic. By the time we reach work we have already been exposed to feelings of anxiety, and immediately remind ourselves of how much work we have to do, taking the word 'busy', and wearing it around our necks like a badge of honour.

Being 'busy' is not something to be proud of. Being 'productive' is a much nicer way of phrasing it, because when you wake up on a Monday morning and say, 'I have a very productive week ahead', you instantly feel good about what lies before you. If you say, 'I am so busy, I have such a busy schedule', you will find that chases you around all week, and you will become anxious and negative. If you are working too hard, you will be in danger of not taking time out to exercise or eat well. And when you are tired, you will get 'hangry' and 'snackered' and reach for the sugary titbits in the canteen.

It is important to take time out, especially if you have to sit down all day in front of a computer screen. And research has shown that multiple small amounts of exercise during the day far outweigh the benefits of a single hour-long gym session. So switch the lift for the stairwell and mount it like you're braving Everest, or pop out round the block for some fresh air and do some deep breathing along the way. Always try to incorporate some stretches whenever you can – muscles can get bunched up and knotty when we sit in the same position for too long, and ultimately this can lead to bad backs, hips and joint issues. However you choose to break up your day, remember that you always need to incorporate time for yourself.

GET PHYSICAL AU NATUREL

It is no secret that daily exercise provides us with countless benefits both physically and mentally. A lot of research shows that the average westerner is getting a lot less light during the day and being exposed to more light at night. This messes with our circadian rhythms and in turn has consequences for our physical and mental health.

Training outdoors can eliminate stress levels and improve mood significantly. Very often we go from one indoor space (work or home) to the next (the gym) and back home again. Even though we go outdoors to get there, realistically we are simply moving between two indoor spaces.

Switching from an indoor gym to outdoor exercise has been proven to help boost mental health. Taking deep breaths comes more naturally when training outdoors and these deep breaths can also help you to feel a lot more calm and alleviate a busy mind. It's not necessary to run a marathon to feel these benefits; simply walking briskly through the park, incorporating some step-ups on a park bench or jogging up some outdoor steps will do the trick.

→ SWITCH TIPS ←

- By its very nature, the word 'stress' is stressful. Switch the word out and instead use something fun and trivial, like funky or squashy.

- Stress in high doses is not only counter-productive; it can also mess with your health. Imagine a glass of stirred salty water slowly stopping swirling. By the time it has settled, your pattern interrupt should have somewhat silenced your stress (yes, I know that's a lot of Ss!)

- Breathe. A basic function, I know; but the most vital. So do it more, and do it slowly.

- Switch social media apps to some meditation apps. There are plenty of free or paid-for apps out there, such as Fearne Cotton's 'Happy Place' meditations on Alexa or Calm, Headspace or Unplug.

- Make sure you switch off all screens at least an hour before you go to bed. Blue light can play havoc with your sleep patterns.

- Switch the word 'busy' to 'productive'. You will find this simple word change will reframe how you view your schedule, and your work-life balance will be more stable.

- Take time out and incorporate multiple shorter workouts, stretches or movements throughout each day. This can be more beneficial than one long workout. Keep moving!

'INSTEAD OF EXERCISING
BECAUSE YOU THINK IT WILL
MAKE YOU *LOOK* GOOD,
EXERCISE BECAUSE IT WILL
MAKE YOU *FEEL* GOOD.'

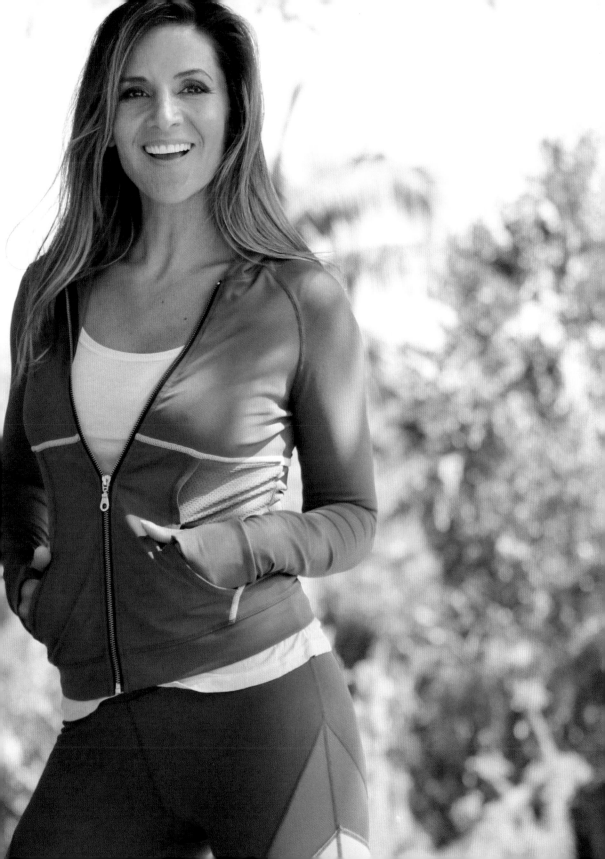

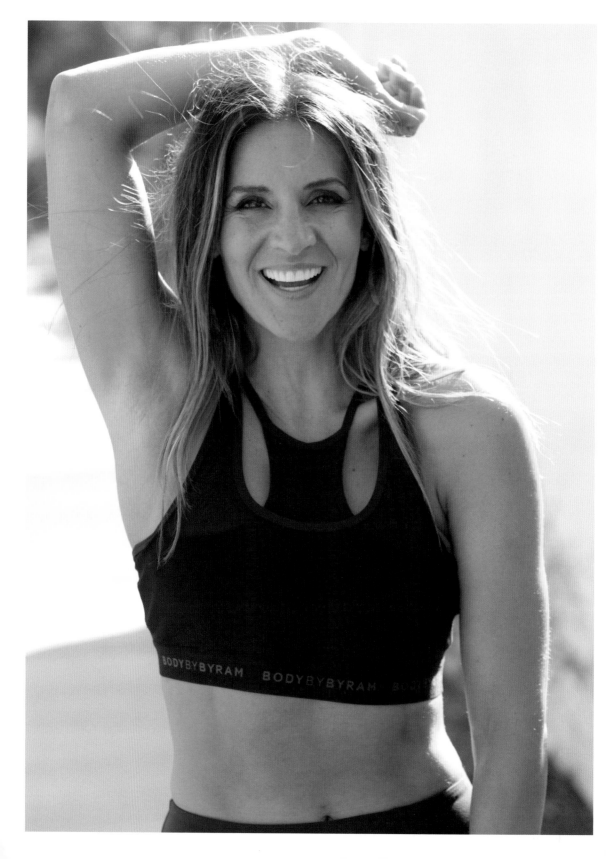

THE
PHILOSOPHY
OF EXERCISE

←——→

WOULDN'T LIFE BE DULL if we all did the same thing all the time? Take exercise, for example. The world would be a pretty boring place if there were one stock solution for getting fit and we simply had to mindlessly repeat routines without tailoring activities to our individual bodies, minds and daily rhythms. There would be no innovation, no interpretation and certainly no joy from discovering new ways to walk, run, stretch, hop, skip or jump.

There are of course some universal truths when it comes to exercise: we should all engage in some type of activity that gets our hearts pumping, blood flowing and muscles working one way or another, pretty much every day. How you do that is entirely up to you, yet before you can begin a lifelong romance with exercise it is important to embrace the underlying reasons why physical activity is so important for our bodies, minds and spirits. So why does it feel so hard sometimes?

Put simply, humans are lazy. And that is not an insult, because we are! It's an evolutionary hangover we can't seem to shake off and by our very nature we have been programmed to conserve energy whenever possible. Think of our prehistoric ancestors for a moment. When they weren't foraging for food or hunting woolly mammoths, they would have been sitting around for large portions of the day, saving their super sauce for the next time there was a rumbling in their bellies or in the bushes. In other words, the Flintstones equivalent of 'Netflix-and-chill' was helpful for their survival and therefore the urge to veg out on the couch often seems so strong, because ... it's in your DNA, girl!

Now, of course I am not telling you this so that you can latch onto it and make the 'lazy is in my DNA' excuse every time someone asks you to join them for a walk. In fact, it is quite the opposite. These days we have it SO easy that between convenience supermarkets, sugary snacks and Deliveroo, we barely have to lift a finger let alone fight and forage to find food – we could literally spend our entire lives sitting on the couch waiting to be fed.

To combat this, we have had to invent ways to recreate the physical rigours of a life around the campfire to burn off those excess calories. So while your great, great, great, great, great grandmother wouldn't have gone to a Sapiens Soul Cycle spin class or headed out to Cavewoman Cross Fit, it is vital that every day, in some way or another, you get up and get going.

Wherever you look, the benefits of exercise are well-documented, from the prevention of illness and prolonged life to mental clarity and improved self-esteem. However, *how* we exercise is not nearly as important as *why* we exercise, so instead of giving you a list of dos and don'ts which you can easily find online, on shelves and on every street corner, I'd like to share with you my golden rules for exercising and the reasons behind them.

DON'T EXERCISE TO LOSE WEIGHT

—

If you have taken anything from the previous pages, I really hope it's that your internal narrative sets the tone for your external experience. Interpreting this for exercise means that if you set out on a fitness journey and tell yourself that weight loss is the be all and end all, then that is all you will focus on. You'll define your success by the numbers on the scales and feel anxious when the little digits don't marry up with your expectations. What's more, you'll miss out on the other benefits of exercise along the way and (here's the scariest part) what happens when you achieve your goal? Lose even more weight? Or maintain skinny, whatever the cost? Let's hope not because I know from personal experience this is a dangerous path to tread that does not lead to long-term life satisfaction.

So instead of exercising because you think it will make you look good, exercise because it will make you feel good ... and when I say feel good, I don't just mean figuratively, because after an hour of intense exercise, not only will your blood be highly oxygenated and your brain be firing on all cylinders, your body will also release pain-relief chemicals called endorphins. As these race around your system, they cause a euphoric feeling comparable to the high experienced from drug taking, which really puts a new spin on the term 'HIIT' training!

That's not to say you should only work out to get a fix of endorphins, which as it happens can be addictive, so be warned. There are so many more reasons to get active than the tiresome bikini body clichés. The benefits are almost endless and you'll feel them a lot sooner than you see them in the mirror.

What's more, when you feel good, you do good and that creates a 360° approach that leads to overall health and happiness. Because a healthy attitude towards exercise is the all-important key. The more you move, the more you rest, meaning you'll sleep more deeply and benefit from more routine sleep patterns. In turn you will wake up feeling refreshed, rested and raring to go again the following day, putting you into a pattern of good lifestyle habits that you can carry out each day without even thinking about it.

BE MINDFUL

—

Don't just rock up to the gym, sit on an exercise bike looking at your phone and expect results once the timer has hit zero. You are in possession of a carefully crafted biomechanical miracle that deserves to do what it was designed to, and it has been designed for you to pay attention while you are doing it. Exercise is about so much more than moving your legs mindlessly; it's about purposeful breathing, careful coordination and learning the language of your body. The more you listen and understand, the more you can speak back. On the other hand, if you are simply going through the motions you'll never develop a rapport with your physical self – surely the most important relationship to nurture. As I said earlier, we humans are lazy and if you are just on auto-pilot, your body will dedicate less and less energy to working out and getting fit.

DON'T BE AFRAID TO TRY SOMETHING NEW

—

Being a novice can be frustrating and often it is easier to turn your back on the possibility of perceived humiliation rather than to get stuck in and see what happens. For example, going into a class can be intimidating, particularly if everyone else seems to know exactly what to do and when to do it. Quite often classes become a little society of their own with unspoken rules, in-jokes and hierarchies that seem confusing, but don't be intimidated and remember that although you might feel foolish, no one is looking at you and rolling their eyes – they are too busy worrying about their own insecurities. You want to go to a dance class? Who cares if you fluff the choreography? You want to try yoga? No one cares if you mix up your downward dog with your child's pose! Your body loves to be pushed in new and different directions, so at least give it a chance.

DON'T BE INTIMIDATED BY THE GYM

—

Many women tell me that they shy away from the weights section at the gym, because it is too male-dominated or because they feel weak and foolish in front of judgemental eyes, especially if they do not know how to use a machine. Well, let me tell you a little bit about the psychology of most gym-goers.

More often than not, gym-goers are in their own world, focusing on their reps and their ability to complete a set. Just like you, they want to get in, work out and get out.

Most gym-goers will be happy to advise you, unless of course they too are navigating unknown territory, in which case you've found a kindred gym spirit! When in training mode, 99.9 per cent of folks at the gym like to be focused on themselves, and therefore, with all due respect, they won't give a rat's arse in hell about your belly, love handles, lack of strength or full-blown female power. Also, the male species of gym-goers thrive on being asked questions and being able to help a damsel in in distress.

If you are still feeling sheepish about entering the weights section, try some of my top tips for getting your mojo on at the gym:

- Find some songs that make you feel POWERFUL. Personally I love anything from '9 to 5' by Dolly to 'Work B**ch' by Britney.
- Blast one of your power-songs in your headphones as you walk into the gym.
- Hold your head up high, keep your back straight, smile and repeat after me (you should know this mantra by now) … 'I am one fucking foxy, funny, fabulous, fit, fantastic, fortuitous female.' Trust me - this will exude some serious energy!

ENJOY IT!

—

Life is too short to spend time doing something you hate, so make sure you find activities you enjoy. What's more, remember that one size does not fit all and what works for those around you might not be the right fit for you. Personally, I don't like swimming. I have tried so many times to get myself into the pool and smash out laps, but I'm not crazy about front crawl, I'm not big on breast stroke, and the less said about the butterfly the better. I have bought specialist snorkels to assist my breathing; I have sought out fancy goggles that minimise the imprint marks on my face and even purchased underwater MP3 players so I can listen to my favourite tunes in a bid to ignore the overwhelming desire to get out and dry off. Yet despite it all, I would rather be doing something else – and that's OK. I know that swimming is a great form of exercise that gets my heart going, my lungs working and muscles moving in a low-impact and supported way, yet the thought of stinking of chlorine, wet hair in winter and aggressive swimming pool lane-hoggers just turns me off.

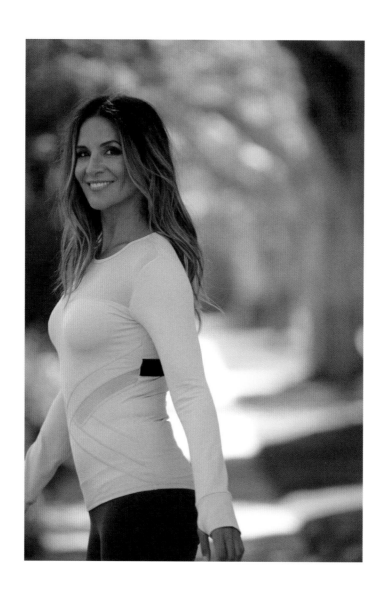

In contrast, my husband loves to swim and says the pool is the one place in the world he can go to mindfully close out the outside world. A place where he is free from phone calls, emails, texts and BBC news updates. He says the churning of the water sends him into a meditative state where he can be creative while getting a serious workout. He has found his lane (pun firmly intended) and that works for him. The point is that you need to find what works for you and embrace it.

CHANGE YOUR MOOD

—

If you aren't in the mood to exercise or you don't feel energetic, take 10 deep breaths and reassess. Deep breathing will oxygenate your body and brain and as few as 10 breaths can be enough to make you feel invigorated, energised and ready to get going. Simply stand with your feet shoulder width apart and exhale, forcing every last ounce of air out of your lungs. Then inhale deeply through your nose, and as your lungs fill, push your tummy out so that your diaphragm lifts and your chest fully inflates. Hold the breath for a moment before forcibly exhaling through your mouth. After 10 breaths, I guarantee you'll feel wide awake and ready for action.

TRY BODYWEIGHT EXERCISES

—

You have your own gym right in front of you: your own bodyweight! Before I talk about the benefits of bodyweight exercises, perhaps now is a good time to discuss what actually happens when you lift weights. First, let's deal with the myth that pumping iron like a terminator will turn you into Arnie. That's just not true and gaining muscle mass at such considerable levels requires a particularly high level of dietary calorie intake and a serious release of muscle-building hormones, such as testosterone, which is naturally much lower in women. When you lift a weight, your muscles will experience micro-tears. These micro-tears in your muscles then heal and grow back leaner if you 'sculpt' them by training the correct way. When you lift weights you will burn calories for longer as your muscles are 'healing' in the aftermath. If weights really are not your cup of tea, then use your body as your weight. There are so many exercises you can do using just your body – such as stationary or jump squats, lunges, push-ups or abdominal crunches.

BE PATIENT

—

We often get impatient when we don't see immediate results, and this can be the ruination of a potentially great fitness journey. It is important to note that when you train, you will not see results immediately. So if you train hard this week, you will not see results until next week or maybe even the week after that. On average, it takes about three weeks before you start to see some serious changes. Take your time and go easy on yourself. You are creating a lifestyle, and that takes time to fall into place.

NO EXCUSES!

—

Saying 'I don't have the time' is simply not an excuse. If you struggle for motivation, consider joining a team. Team sports can be a great way to introduce exercise into your life while simultaneously improving your coordination skills, building mental strength and even presenting new opportunities for sociability outside your existing circle of friends.

Regrettably, most of us leave team sports behind once we finish school, yet it's worth remembering why it was such an important part of the curriculum in our younger years. Beyond the physical benefits, we learned vital lessons about the responsibility of being relied on by others as well as the vulnerability that comes from relying on others to achieve. We meditated by clearing our mind of all the chatter and focusing entirely on the goal, net, racket, ball, puck or shuttlecock.

I understand you might not have the happiest memoires of school sports, linked to things like ill-fitting, scratchy kits and bitchy remarks in the changing rooms, but adult sports teams are different. First, everyone who is there wants to be there, making for a much happier environment. Second, the stakes are much lower, and the FA Cup Final, win-at-all-costs mentality of adolescent sports teams no longer applies. Sure, you'll have to compete, but that's half the fun.

Another reason why amateur sports teams are so good to engage in is that they are geared around a weekly routine with specific times each week for training and matches, allowing players to get into a rhythm that they can block out on their schedules.

Also, remember that the world is your treadmill! If running or walking is your exercise of choice, then all you need is a pair of trainers and a dollop of enthusiasm: simply open your front door and off you go!

BUDDY UP

—

Having a support system is also extremely important. If team games aren't your vibe, it is helpful to find a friend who wants to go on this journey with you. You're only human and willpower can cave, so if you can convince a partner to get on this health kick with you it will make it a lot easier. Also, it makes it far harder to skip your exercise when you know that there might be consequences such as letting someone down (see accountability, page 154).

BANISH GUILT IF YOU MISS A WORKOUT

—

If you miss a workout, or two or three or four, don't worry or beat yourself up. If you are regularly active, you'll be more sensitive to inactivity. Therefore, missing a workout might make you feel agitated and restless. That's OK – it's simply your body reminding you to move. Just make sure you don't burden yourself with guilt for not being active; your body has muscle memory and will snap back into workout mode as soon as you do.

TRAIN SMARTER NOT HARDER

—

Training excessively in the short term can be counterproductive to your long-term goals. Your body will crash and burn and your efforts will not be rewarded because you will be too tired, hungry and grumpy to train like a pro. So train smarter not harder by doing shorter, more intense sessions. Really focus on every move and feel the burn, rather than spending hours wandering around the gym, or scrolling through your phone on the cross trainer.

REST AND RESET

—

Rest days are just as important as training days. It is during these resting periods that your muscles heal and rebuild. So make sure you add in a rest day at least every two to three days. If you are training at the gym consistently and have a productive lifestyle, your muscles will inevitably get tired. Tired muscles lead to injury, which in turn will stop you training and having a productive lifestyle. Vicious cycle, eh? Give your muscles a twice-weekly bath with Epsom salts or magnesium flakes – added bonus: the salts help to eliminate toxins from your body!

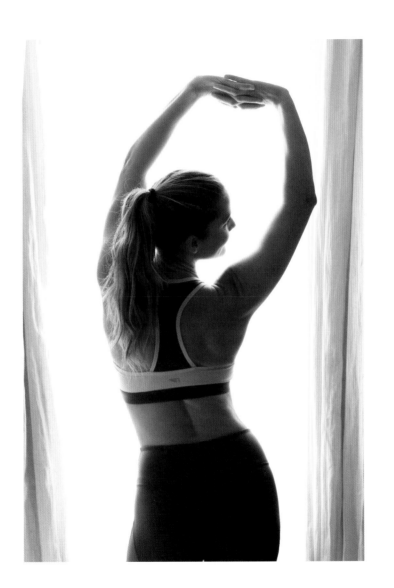

IT'S NEVER TOO LATE TO START

—

If you are reading this in your forties and you spent your twenties lifting pizzas and pints rather than barbells and battle ropes, then please know it is never too late to start your fitness journey. Having said that, the sooner you start the better because muscle memory is formed over years and the best time to instil muscle memory is in our twenties. Better muscle memory means we snap back into shape more easily after long periods of inactivity.

While it *is* harder to start in later life, it is also true that we all have to start somewhere if we truly want positive results. And by doing so NOW, by the time you get to your fifties, sixties, seventies or eighties, you will be grateful for having jumped on that fabulous, fun and foxy fitness wagon.

One really important reason to get motivated is that as we age, we lose lean mass (about 5lb per decade) made up of mostly muscle and bone. This would suggest that our metabolic decline isn't about our actual age per se, rather the choices we make about our lifestyle. It may or may not come as a surprise to you then that when we think of 'ageing', it isn't about the number, but inactivity and bad dietary decisions. More still, this means that while we cannot rewind the clock or the number of candles on our birthday cakes, we CAN be in charge of our body's ageing process! Eating well and exercising to look after our muscles mean that we can age more slowly, and be feisty and fit much later in life.

→ SWITCH TIPS ←

- Exercise! It will make you feel good and when you feel good, you do good.

- If you are going to work out, put your heart into it. Don't dilly-dally. Get in, get it done and get out.

- Try new things – you never know what you might enjoy.

- Switch gym weights for bodyweight exercises such as lunging, squatting and push-ups if you can't get to a gym.

- Be patient. Remember, your hard work does not show immediately. Be consistent and the results will eventually show.

- You are stronger than your excuses.

- Make sure you have some rest days and treat your body to some down time.

- Train in pairs or join a team, if that's a good incentive. People are always looking for company, so make it a social occasion.

- If you miss a workout or two, don't worry about it. Just get back to it when you can. Your body has muscle memory; it knows how to snap back.

- It's never too late to start this journey.

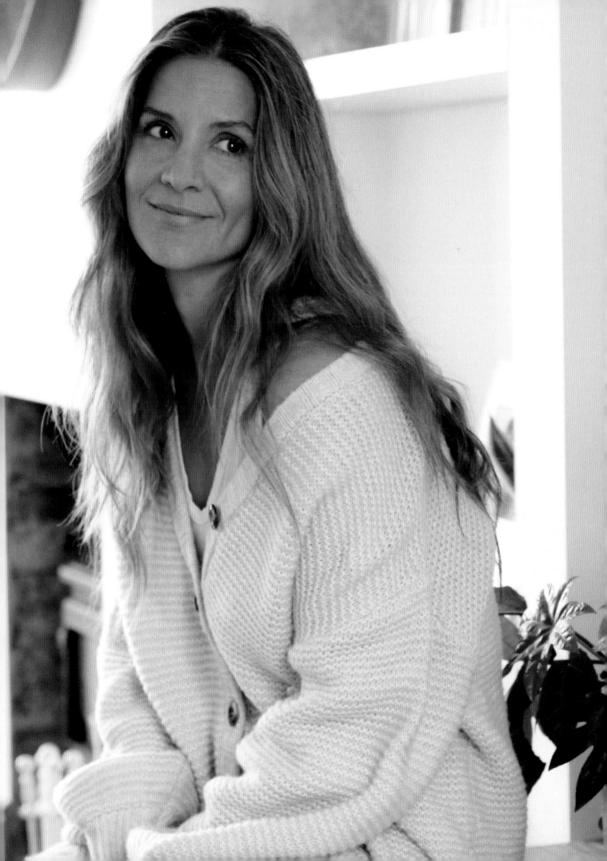

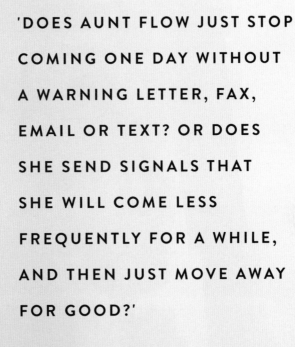

'DOES AUNT FLOW JUST STOP
COMING ONE DAY WITHOUT
A WARNING LETTER, FAX,
EMAIL OR TEXT? OR DOES
SHE SEND SIGNALS THAT
SHE WILL COME LESS
FREQUENTLY FOR A WHILE,
AND THEN JUST MOVE AWAY
FOR GOOD?'

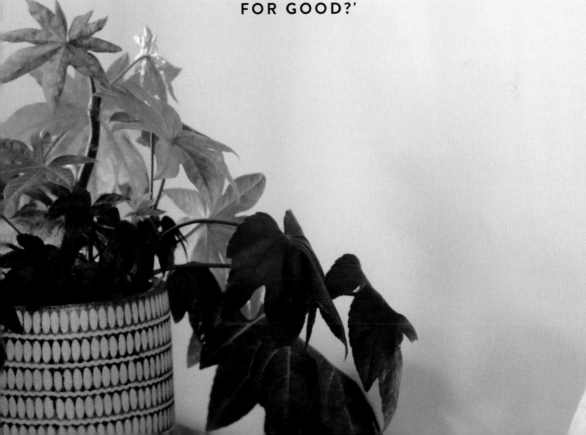

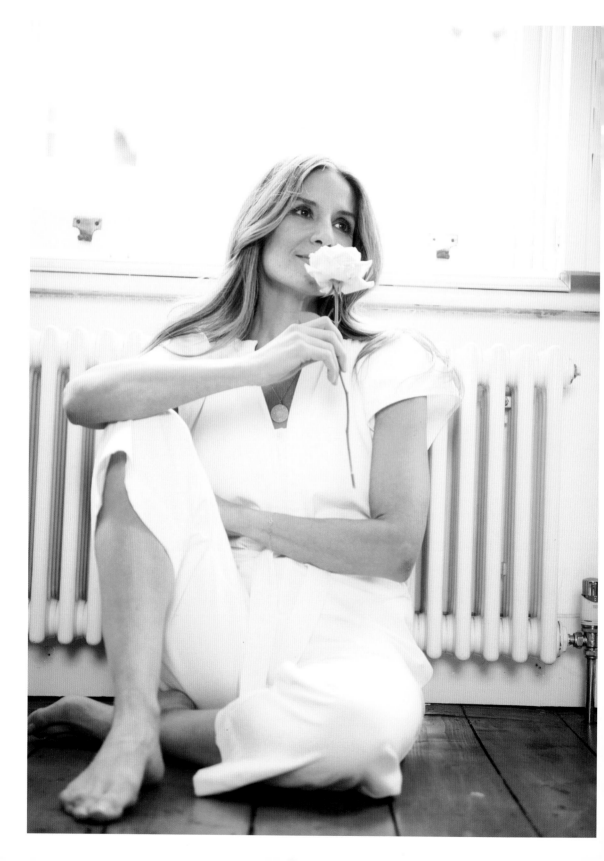

THE
BIG PAUSE

⟵⟶

PERSONALLY I HAVE YET to experience the menopause; 'yet' being the operative word here, because the menopause is an unavoidable (and a very natural) part of the female ageing process. So, to be prepared, it is important to be bright-eyed, bushy-tailed and fully aware of what lies ahead on the road to the Big Pause.

In the most literal sense the word 'menopause' is taken from the Greek words 'mēn' and 'pausis', meaning month and pause. But does Aunt Flow just stop coming one day without a warning letter, fax, email or text? Or does she send signals that she will come less frequently for a while, and then just move away for good? And what are the implications of not having any more periods? Is it simply that we can rejoice at the thought of never having to buy tampons again, or does the menopause come with extra added emotions, feelings and physical effects?

The simple answer is that it will vary from woman to woman, from little to no symptoms, to life-altering changes. The menopause can kick in anywhere between the ages of 45 to 55, so on average women tend to experience it by age 51.

But even before the paint shop gets shut for good, we can expect to go through a phase called perimenopause, or peri as I will call it for short. Understanding what this involves can help you prepare for the real thing.

Peri can take place over a period (pardon the pun) of several years, even as early as 10 years before Aunt Flow finally packs her bags for good. This phase is the run-up, the pre-game or the foreplay to the Big Pause, and it is during this time that our ovaries are gradually rebalancing their oestrogen and progesterone production to prepare for the main event.

Now, just because you still have your period, that doesn't mean you are not in peri. This fact causes confusion among many women who wrongly assume that symptoms of the menopause only appear after periods stop.

There are also many cases of early menopause; for some people, peri can kick in by the late thirties. Let's take an example: have you ever had months when you had an unexplained 'missed period' and knew for hella sure you were not pregnant because, well, you 'had a headache' all month. These can be explained as 'anovulatory cycles', and can be a possible sign that peri has kicked in.

The menopause is a completely natural, normal and gradual process and not a 'disease' to be treated. Nevertheless, it is important to buckle up and get ready, ladies, because no matter what age you get there, being prepared is the key to a happy farewell to Aunt Flow.

SOME (DON'T) LIKE IT HOT

—

Hot flushes happen as a result of hormonal fluctuations, usually experienced as feelings of sudden heat in the face, neck and chest, sometimes resulting in red and sweaty skin. Like everything else, these can differ from one woman to the next, but more than 80 per cent of women can be burdened by hot flushes at some point during peri or menopause. Symptoms can start long before your period stops and can continue for several years afterwards.

TO HELP: The moment you feel a flush coming on, stop what you're doing, take some deep breaths and try to chill, and if you can, drink some cold water. In general, eating small, regular meals can also help because the process of digesting a large meal can generate heat and sometimes bring on a flush. If you smoke – QUIT! Research shows that smoking can increase the severity of hot flushes.

SWEATY BETTY

—

Night sweats are hot flushes that take place at night. They can understandably leave you feeling tired and generally pooped (and with damp bed sheets and nightwear to wash the next morning).

TO HELP: Cool your bedroom at night by leaving a window ajar or using a fan and always have a towel by your bed. Having water on hand is also a good idea, so you can cool down and rehydrate from all the lost fluids. Try changing to cotton sheets and nightwear, or better still, sleep naked. Hot flushes can be exacerbated by caffeine, alcohol and some spicy foods, so cut back or eliminate these if you can.

CAN'T SLEEP, WON'T SLEEP

—

Insomnia is one of the most common signs of the Big Pause, although it's no surprise that it's hard to sleep if you're plagued by night sweats.

TO HELP: Make sure to avoid stimulants if you are experiencing trouble sleeping – that mid-afternoon coffee or those late-night glasses of wine will not do your sleep patterns any favours. Try replacing them with calming herbal tea such as chamomile tea, sleepy tea, or a hot soya milk drink (soya contains isoflavones that can help to regulate oestrogen levels).

Also, try avoiding blue light and TV before bed, as they will make it harder to fall asleep (see page 172). Lack of sleep will affect your mood the next day, so the sooner you get your sleep patterns in check, the better. If sleepless nights are common, make sure you take your 40 winks whenever you can, without a smidgen of guilt.

MOODY MARE

—

Mood swings and a change from your usual temperament can be a sign of peri and menopause as your hormones peak and trough like a rollercoaster. If you find yourself in tears at the latest episode of *Neighbours*, you might want to take note of the frequency that you are reaching for the Kleenex. Feelings of anxiety and panic are also signs that you are going through menopause, so be aware and mindful to give yourself a break if these feelings are occurring more and more often.

TO HELP: Try to use some meditation techniques that we discussed in the Zen chapter (see page 165). Plus, getting outdoors and exercising is a great way to tackle the blues if you can (see page 174).

DRY AS THE SAHARA DESERT

—

As ladies age, oestrogen levels plummet, meaning less lubrication during sexy time. Half of women will experience vaginal dryness (oh, the joys) during menopause and no matter how many Ryan Reynolds movies you watch, this lack of sexy juice can lead to lack of arousal and, if left unattended, can put a real dampener on your sex life.

TO HELP: Don't let this put you off having sex. Ironically, regular sex can actually help vaginal lubrication, as can foreplay. Start supplying your body with naturally occurring oestrogen through your diet by regularly consuming soya products and flax seeds. Taking a daily supplement such as sea buckthorn can also help your body produce the cells that create lubrication.

STOP THE BUS, I WANT TO WEE-WEE!

—

In general, a decreased ability to hold urine can happen after having babies, during menopause or once you hit your forties (Hurrah!) This happens because the elasticity and tone of the vaginal wall decreases with age. So if you have ever been in a situation where you haven't quite made it to the loo on time – instead of reaching for the adult nappies, try the below.

TO HELP: Doing regular pelvic floor exercises can really help to strengthen the muscles in the vagina so your pee doesn't come out quite so easily! These are called Kegel exercises and involve simply tensing the muscles you would use to stop yourself peeing, then releasing. A good way to do this is to start and stop your urine flow several times while urinating.

NOT TONIGHT, LOVE, I'VE (REALLY) GOT A HEADACHE

—

Headaches and migraines are common during the menopause and may be the result of fluctuating body temperature, hot flush exhaustion, sleeplessness or general stress and anxiety.

TO HELP: Try to incorporate anti-inflammatories such as ginger and turmeric into your diet and avoid caffeine and alcohol where possible.

SCALY SKIN

—

Many women notice their skin becoming drier around the time of the menopause. This can be a direct effect of lack of oestrogen levels. Apart from getting natural oestrogen in your diet, try to re-evaluate your skincare regime.

TO HELP: Regularly exfoliate your skin and add a good oil or serum to your skincare habits. Make sure to wear a good SPF if you are braving the sun and get some extra hydration by drinking lots of water. Also, foods rich in omega-3 fats will help to keep skin soft and smooth.

MY ACHY, ACHY JOINTS

—

Believe it or not, stiff and aching joints and creaking bones as you get out of bed might be caused by a lack of oestrogen.

TO HELP: Getting your five-a-day, omega-3s, and embarking on regular exercise can alleviate these symptoms. Make sure you get your vitamin D levels tested: a deficiency can be the cause of aching bones. Also, vitamin K is a very important addition to your diet to get calcium into your bones; when taken with vitamin D it can have even more impressive results.

EAT RIGHT

—

Eating the right food is crucial when it comes to alleviating symptoms of menopause.

TO HELP:

- Take **FISH OIL SUPPLEMENTS** or add oily fish (such as salmon or mackerel) to a meal to balance the hormones oestrogen and progesterone.
- Phytoestrogens such as isoflavones help to balance hormones naturally and can be found in vegetables such as **BROCCOLI, KOHLRABI, PAK CHOI** and **RADISHES**.
- Other hormone-balancing substances called lignans can be found in **BEANSPROUTS, CHICKPEAS, SWEET POTATOES, LENTILS** and **SEEDS** (flax seed and pumpkin seeds are the best choices).
- Don't forget soya products — **SOYA MILK** and **SOYA YOGHURTS** are good ways to increase your intake.
- Foods high in fibre such as **WHOLEGRAINS, PULSES** and **VEGETABLES** help to lower cholesterol (which can rise in menopausal women) and control weight fluctuations (another side-effect some women experience).

MOVE

—

Exercise is important for ladies as we get older, and just because strength naturally declines and muscle mass is lost that does not mean you can't combat it. Studies show that resistance (weight) training can actually reverse the ageing process at a genetic level. In our forties our bodies become less efficient at producing and releasing key hormones responsible for many important body functions, and weight/strength training regulates the release of many hormones. This means that we can stabilise insulin levels, blood sugar can be regulated, and in general the effects of ageing are slowed down. Also, remember that the hormone testosterone allows for the upkeep of muscle mass, so step into that weights section, girls (see page 182).

To sum up, the best way to prepare for this particular journey is to take regular exercise and maintain a healthy weight, reduce or stop smoking, limit alcohol and caffeine intake and stay as calm as possible. The sooner you make your changes, the easier 'the change' and the years beyond will be.

'MOST OF ALL, ENJOY WHAT YOU MAKE AND TREAT EVERY MEAL LIKE A GIFT TO YOUR INCREDIBLE BODY.'

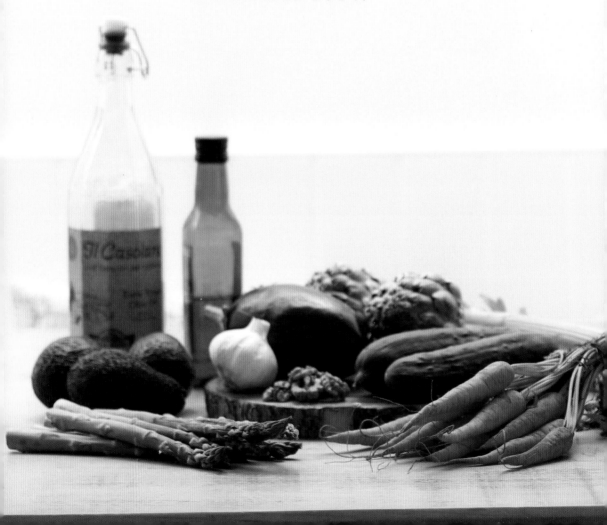

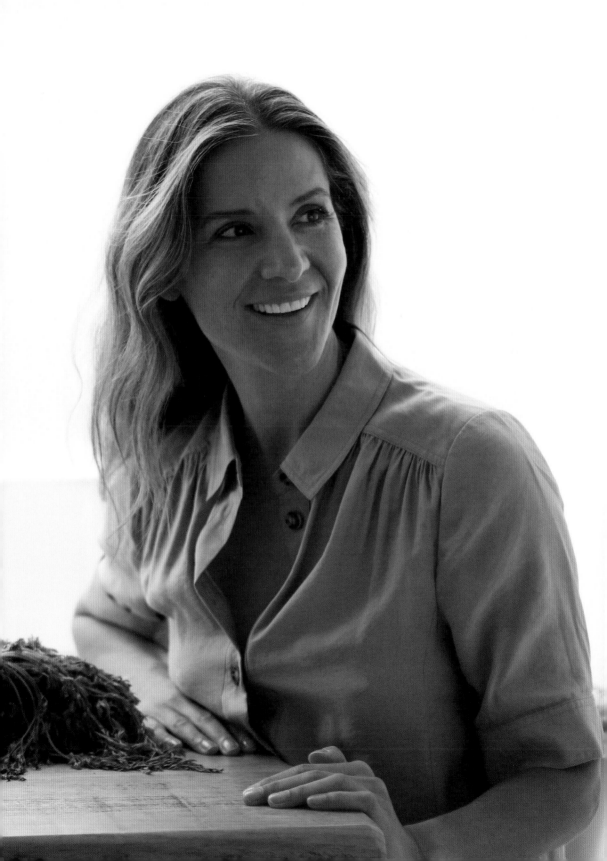

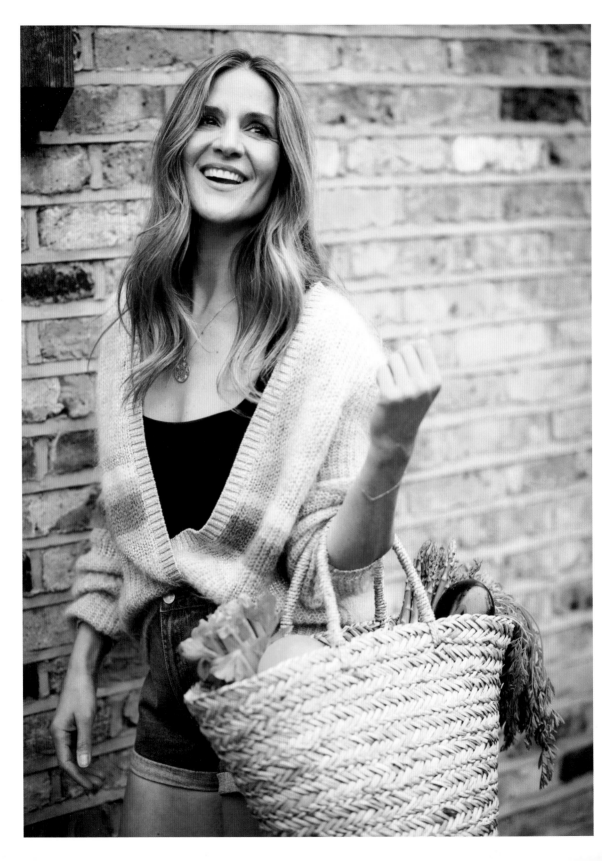

FOOD
FOR THOUGHT:
RECIPES

$\longleftrightarrow$

I BELIEVE IN KEEPING food simple yet tasty. I understand that most of you, like me, have productive lives, which often cause us to rush our meals and cook without thought or consideration. So my top trick is to always keep ingredients simple, keep cooking relatively hassle-free, plan ahead and prepare meals in advance when possible. Most of all, enjoy what you make and treat every meal like a gift to your incredible body. Before we get into recipes, it's important to understand the philosophies of eating well. My food philosophy is based on four things: unprocessed food, cooking well, good-quality ingredients and food preparation.

UNPROCESSED FOOD

—

If it grows on the land, swims, eats grass or flies, you are good to go. Try to stay away from anything that is too far away from its original form: if it has a label on it with a lot of ingredients, then you probably shouldn't be eating it.

COOK WELL

—

Cooking from scratch is always better than heating up foods bought in plastic containers. This does take longer, so try to put a few minutes aside each day to prepare. In general, stir-frying, grilling, sautéing, baking, barbecuing and steaming are better choices than frying or microwaving.

GOOD-QUALITY INGREDIENTS

—

Whenever possible, look for grass-fed meats, organic or free range poultry and wild fish. This way you have less chance of eating toxins and steroids that a lot of less sustainabe products contain. In addition, nutritionally dense food will satisfy you for longer, and the more food you can eat that is serving your body on a cellular level, the less your body will crave sugary foods.

ADVANCE FOOD PREPARATION

—

Make good choices, before the only choice you have is a bad one. Good, whole foods will not be available in a lot of places you go such as the canteen at work, an airport or aeroplane or the beach. You cannot rely on restaurants or a shop to have a stock of your essentials. If you don't have time every day, prep on a Sunday for the week ahead. Make a large pot of brown rice or quinoa, boil six eggs, chop raw veggies, and steam or grill a few pieces of salmon or chicken. Put them all into separate Tupperware boxes and pop in the fridge (be sure to cool the rice completely first). Next, get five clean jam jars and make overnight oatmeal, and mix a handful of nuts and goji berries in Ziploc bags for snacking on the go. Et voilà! You have a week's worth of food in advance ready to go.

AMANDA'S CUPBOARD AND
FRIDGE ESSENTIALS

—

GRAINS

- Oatmeal
- Quinoa
- Brown rice

- Wholewheat pasta
- Rice/corn cakes

- Dark breads such as wholewheat or rye

SEEDS

- Sunflower seeds

- Pumpkin seeds

- Sesame seeds (black)

VEG

- Green veg: kale, spinach, broccoli, asparagus

- Root veg: carrots, sweet potatoes, white potatoes, beetroots, onions, parsnips, sugar snap peas, peas (fresh or frozen), runner beans, green beans

- Salad: peppers, cucumber, radishes, spring onions, mushrooms, celery

FRUITS

- Bananas
- Grapefruit
- Oranges
- Avocados
- Tomatoes
- Apples

- Dark berries such as blueberries and blackberries
- Aubergines
- Kiwis
- Lemons and limes

- Dried berries that are high in antioxidants: goji berries, mulberries, golden berries

MEATS AND FISH

- Fish: salmon, sea bass, prawns, scallops, cod, trout

- Meat: turkey, chicken, chicken livers, pork, lean organic red meat (such as beef and lamb)

NUTS (UNROASTED AND UNSALTED)

- Almonds
- Cashews

- Brazil nuts
- Pine nuts

- Walnuts
- Coconut flakes

VEGAN/VEGETARIAN SOURCES OF PROTEIN

- Tofu

- Tempeh
- Edamame beans

- Protein powder (vegan if possible)

HERBS, SPICES AND FLAVOURINGS

- Cinnamon
- Turmeric powder
- Ginger
- Garlic

- Basil
- Tarragon
- Parsley
- Mint

- Thyme
- Dill

CONDIMENTS

- Honey mustard
- Tahini
- Agave syrup/coconut nectar

- Balsamic vinegar
- Nut butters
- Himalayan salt
- Sea salt

- Black pepper
- Vanilla extract
- Bragg Liquid Aminos

OILS

- Olive oil

- Coconut oil

- Rapeseed oil

PULSES

- Lentils
- Garden peas

- Chickpeas
- Butter beans

- Kidney beans
- Cannellini beans

SUPERFOODS

- Chia seeds
- Maca powder
- Matcha green tea powder
- Baobab powder
- Cacao – nibs and powder
- Flax seeds
- Bee pollen
- Hemp seeds

FRIDGE ESSENTIALS

- Eggs
- Yoghurt (vegan/Greek)
- Vegetable broth
- Tomato purée
- Cottage cheese
- Milks – almond, cashew, oat, rice, soya, goat's, sheep's or cow's (full fat)

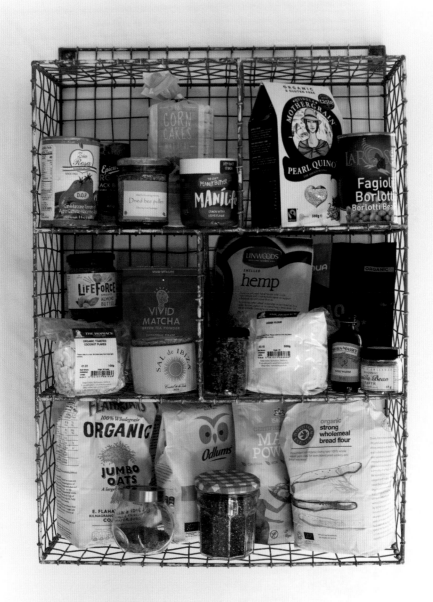

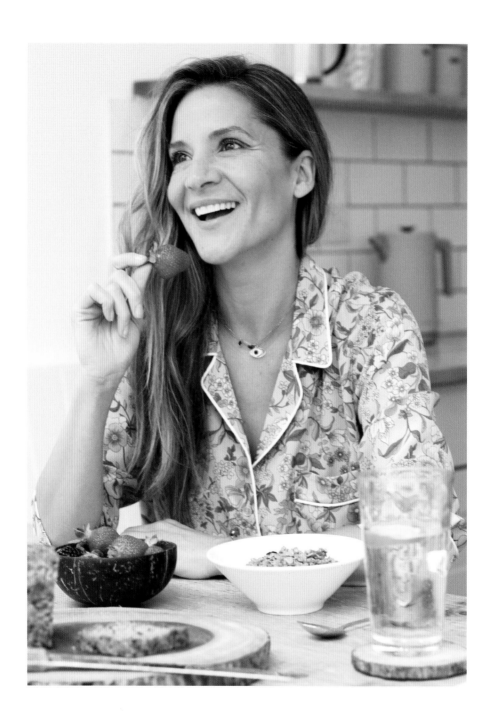

BREAKFAST

—

I want to talk about breakfast in detail because bad habits formed at the start of your day can have monumental consequences for not just the day ahead, but also for your body, mind, skin, moods and general health long-term. Breakfast is often considered the most important meal of the day because it sets your energy levels up for the coming hours, whatever they may hold – whether it's a meeting, an exercise class, a lecture or the school run. Having breakfast, even a small one, kick-starts your metabolism and sends a signal to your brain that it is time to wake up and get going. Yet more often than not it is the most neglected meal, with many of us 'grabbing and going' to get out the door.

BREAKFAST MISTAKES

- Eating food low in nutrients.
- Eating little to no protein or fat.
- Eating foods high in fast carbs (sugar). The sugary content spikes our blood sugar levels, leaving us on a peak-and-crash rollercoaster all day.

THE BIG BREAKFAST OFFENDERS

- **SUGARY CEREALS** – almost all are highly processed, even some of the 'healthy, wholegrain' ones. They are a perfect example of a breakfast that is high in carbohydrates and low in protein and healthy fats, certain to give you a sugary high followed by a crash. Avoid boxed cereals as much as you can: if the packaging boasts that they contain vitamins and minerals, these are most likely synthetic nutrients added back in after processing.

- **CROISSANTS OR MUFFINS** – these are almost always made with white, refined flour. White flour is stripped of most of its minerals and vitamins, meaning it is quickly recognised by the body as sugar and absorbed. Again, the absence of any good-quality protein or fat mean that this process is not slowed down, and the rate of absorption when the sugar hits your system is much faster. Faster high = faster crash.

- Excess **COFFEE** laden with sweeteners and high in saturated fat (see The Great Caffeine Debate on page 65).

- **SUGAR-PACKED FRUIT JUICES** – I know, yes, fruit *is* healthy. However, do not be fooled into thinking that commercially made fruit 'juice' is good for you. In fact, it has been stripped of the fibre that enables the absorption of the sugar to be modified and slowed down. For example, a 300ml glass of juice contains around 25 grams of sugar – that's about SIX teaspoons. And remember, there is no fat or protein to slow the rate of this absorption down, so it is like an IV drip of pure sugar into your system. Especially avoid fruit juices 'from concentrate', because these are heavily processed and often contain extra sugar and almost none of the vitamins, minerals and healthy antioxidants that you would find in fresh fruit.

- **'LOW-FAT' FOODS** – don't be fooled; the fat in these products is just replaced with sugar to make them taste good.

All these high-calorie foods, particularly processed ones, are more likely to contain 'empty calories' and be high in refined carbohydrates but low in the other nutritional components needed to keep your body functioning effectively.

$\longrightarrow$ **SWITCH TIPS** $\longleftarrow$

- Switch the time of your first coffee to 15 minutes later. If you are dehydrated (which most of us are after a sleep) drinking coffee can potentially bring your metabolism to a halt: that's no way to start the day.

- Instead, start your day with oodles of water. As soon as I wake up I drink a big glass of warm water laced with apple cider vinegar (the one that has friendly bacteria called the 'mother'). The warm water wakes up your vital organs, helps to flush toxins out of your system and re-hydrates you. The vinegar helps aid digestion, boosts energy and helps keep blood sugar levels balanced, which is exactly what you need first thing in the morning. That should stop you running for the sugary muffin.

- Switch plain water to lemon water (especially if you don't fancy the vinegar). Lemons are alkalising (they are acidic on their own, but once the body metabolises them they are alkaline) and an alkaline body is one we are aiming for – the opposite is acidic, and that's where disease can thrive.

- Try to eat within an hour of waking so you can rev up your metabolism rather than starve your body. Your metabolism is at its most efficient in the morning so make use of it! Your body doesn't like to be starved, and because it is clever it will start clinging to things and storing them as fat if it thinks it is going into starvation mode.

- Stay away from 'sweet' breakfasts as much as you can. Teach your taste buds to 'start as you mean to go on' for the day. Adding greens, such as spinach, will do the trick.

- Switch high-sugar breakfast foods to things like:
  - Eggs and avocado on rye toast
  - Oatmeal with cashew nut milk topped with seeds and berries
  - Salmon on rye toast
  - Homemade granola
  - Oatcakes with nut butter
  - Full-fat yoghurt or coconut yoghurt with seeds and berries
  - Green juices and smoothies with fresh fruit, not concentrated fruit juice.

EGG-SELENT WHITE OMELETTE

—

SERVES 1

- 3 egg whites
- 1 tsp coconut oil
- ½ a thumb-sized piece of fresh ginger, peeled and finely chopped
- a handful of cherry tomatoes
- 1 tsp mild chilli powder
- a large handful of fresh spinach
- ½ an avocado, peeled and sliced
- a slice of rye toast or corn cakes
- olive oil
- a pinch of Himalayan salt

Gently whisk the egg whites in a bowl. In a small non-stick pan, heat the oil and add in the ginger, cherry tomatoes and chilli powder.

Add in the spinach and stir until wilted. Tip in the eggs and leave on a low heat until cooked to your liking. Flip the omelette (or leave it as a scramble if you prefer).

Serve with sliced avocado and a slice of rye toast or corn cakes. Drizzle over some olive oil and sprinkle with some salt.

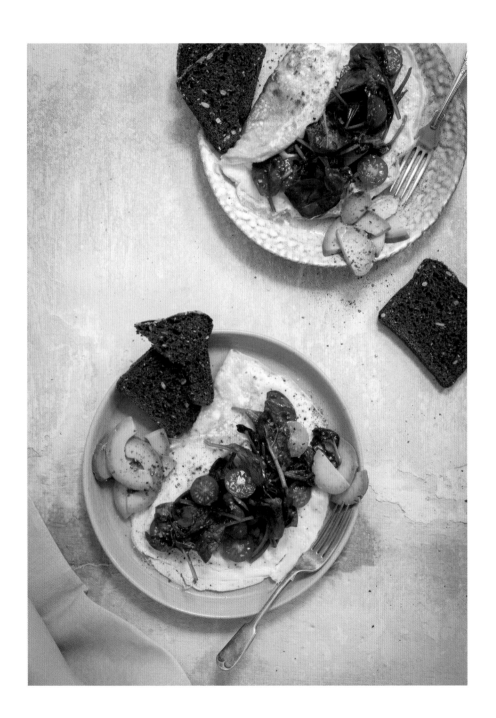

PROTEIN PANCAKES

—

MAKES APPROXIMATELY 3 PANCAKES

- 3 egg whites
- 'flour' of choice: 1 scoop whey protein powder/ sprouted wholegrain rice protein or 30g coconut flour
- 1 tsp vanilla extract
- 2 tbsp almond milk
- 1 tsp agave syrup or manuka honey
- 1 tsp ground cinnamon
- 1 tbsp ground flax seeds
- ¼ banana, peeled and mashed
- a handful of berries (fresh berries or dried goji berries or mulberries are fine)
- coconut oil (for frying)

TO SERVE:
- 2 strawberries, sliced, or a handful of blueberries
- 1 tbsp Greek or coconut yoghurt (optional)

Whisk up all the batter ingredients in a bowl.

Dollop scoops of the mixture into a non-stick pan that has a small amount of coconut oil heated on medium.

Cook until golden on both sides.

Top with sliced strawberries or a sprinkle of blueberries. Dollop on some yoghurt if you like.

SWITCH TIP
These contain your protein and fibre hit, without dairy or gluten. Not only are they perfect for breakfast, they make a great post-workout meal.

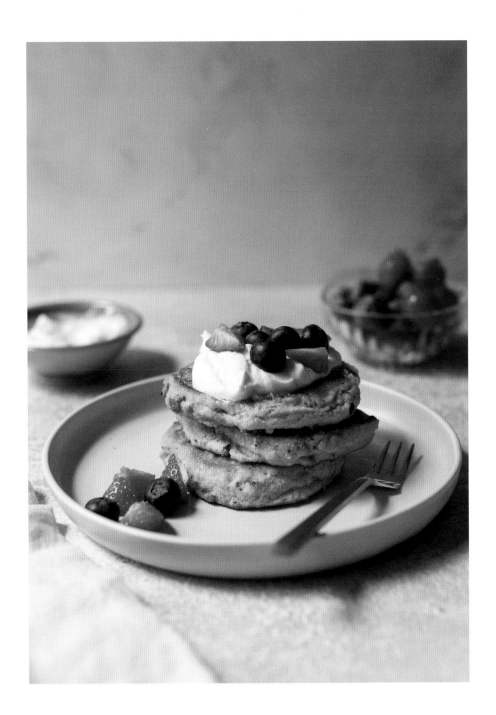

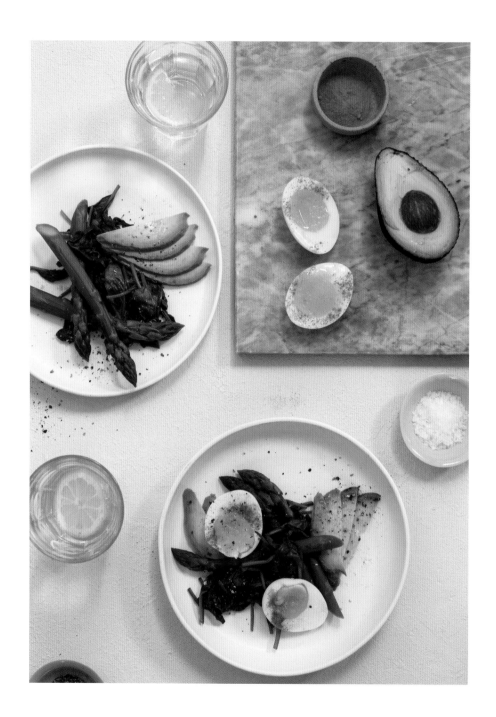

SAUTÉED GREENS WITH EGGS

—

SERVES 2

- 2 eggs
- 200g spinach
- 6 asparagus tips
- olive oil
- a sprinkle of ground turmeric
- ½ an avocado, peeled and chopped
- some cooked sweet potato, cut into cubes (optional; if you have leftovers)

Boil the eggs to a consistency of your liking and leave aside to cool. Sauté the spinach and asparagus in a pan with a little olive oil.

Peel and chop up the boiled eggs, and sprinkle some turmeric on top.

Divide the sautéed spinach and asparagus between two plates, then layer over the eggs, chopped avocado and sweet potato (if using).

AMANDA'S SUPER PORRIDGE

—

SERVES 1

- 50g oats (gluten-free if needed)
- 250ml liquid of choice (water, almond, oat, cashew or coconut milk, goat's/sheep's milk)
- 1 tsp almond butter/nut butter of choice
- 1 tbsp flax seeds
- 1 tsp chia seeds
- 2 tbsp goji berries
- 2 tbsp sunflower and/or pumpkin seeds
- 2 tbsp coconut flakes, toasted in a dry pan
- ½ an apple, grated

OPTIONAL EXTRAS:
- a pinch of grated orange zest
- 1 tsp hemp seeds (for an extra protein boost)

TO SERVE:
- 1 tbsp cacao nibs
- a pinch of cinnamon powder

Put all the ingredients for the porridge in a medium-sized saucepan and cook on a medium heat for about 8 minutes, stirring regularly. Stir in the cacao nibs and cinnamon or sprinkle them on top.

SWITCH TIP
This porridge on its own packs a punch, full of vitamins, nutrients and superfoods, but you can add ½ a scoop of protein powder when it's cooking, or a boiled egg on the side. Protein will keep you fuller for longer.

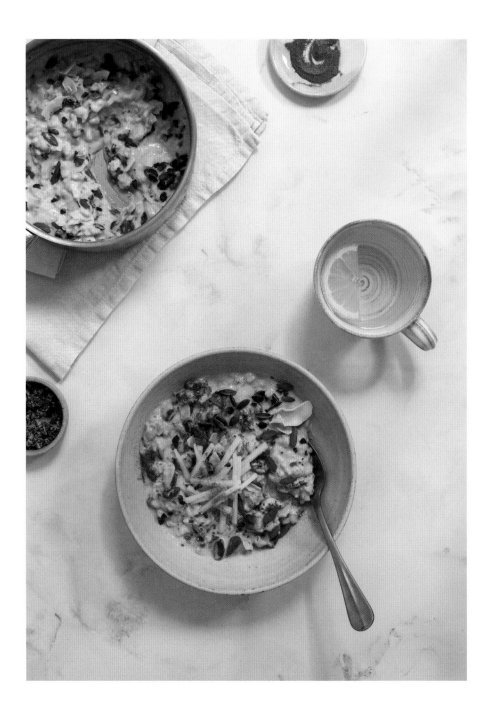

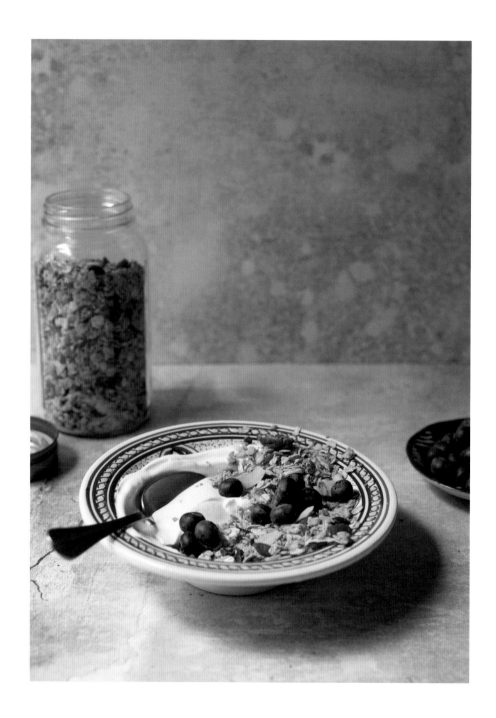

HOMEMADE GRANOLA

—

MAKES ABOUT 500G (ABOUT THE SIZE OF A BOX OF SHOP-BOUGHT CEREAL)

- 2½ tbsp coconut oil
- 2 tbsp coconut nectar or agave syrup
- 400g gluten-free oats
- 3 tbsp nuts of your choice, such as almonds
- 3 tbsp seeds of choice, such as pumpkin and/or sunflower
- 60g coconut flakes
- a handful of dried goji, golden or mulberries (or some of each)
- 1 tsp ground cinnamon
- 3 tbsp cacao nibs

Melt 2 tablespoons of coconut oil in a large sauté pan over a medium heat. Add either the coconut nectar or agave syrup.

Tip in the gluten-free oats and stir well to fully coat the oats in the mixture, allowing them to toast slightly. Spread them out over the bottom of the pan and keep on a low heat, toasting. Be careful not to let this burn while you get on with the rest of the recipe.

In another large, wide pan, melt the rest of the coconut oil and stir in the nuts and seeds, followed by the coconut flakes and dried berries of choice. Sprinkle over the cinnamon and continue to stir until toasted.

Once the mixture is looking golden and toasty, add in your crispy oats from the other pan and mix everything together.

Allow your granola to cool down before stirring through the cacao nibs.

SWITCH TIP
This is a fantastic breakfast choice for a few reasons: oats are a slow-release carb, so you get sustained energy for longer. And cacao nibs have more antioxidants than any plant food on Earth! That makes for a GREAT start to your day!

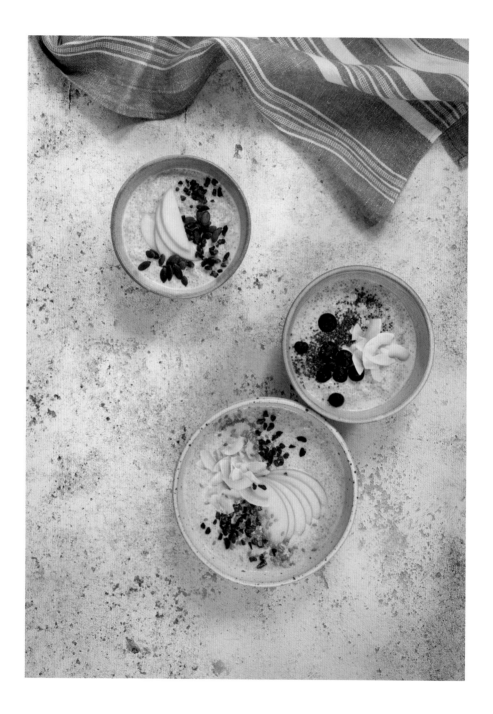

QUINOA PORRIDGE

—

SERVES 1

TO COOK THE QUINOA:
- 180g quinoa
- 1 tsp coconut oil
- 500ml boiling water

TO MAKE THE PORRIDGE:
- water or nut milk as desired, warmed
- a small handful of nuts (cashews, almonds or hazelnuts)
- ½ a chopped apple
- a sprinkle of coconut flakes
- 1 tsp chia seeds
- a sprinkle of sunflower/pumpkin seeds
- 1 tbsp cacao nibs
- a small handful of blueberries

To make quinoa, wash it in a sieve and, in a saucepan, shallow fry the water off with the coconut oil.

Once all the residual water from washing has been fried off, add 500ml of boiling water. Bring back to the boil and simmer for about 15 minutes, by which time this water should have boiled off.

Remove from the heat, cover, and set aside for five minutes to steam, until fluffy. This will make around 3 cups of cooked quinoa, so reserve two-thirds and store, airtight, in the fridge for up to a week to use in other recipes.

To make the quinoa porridge, put a cup of cooked quinoa in a bowl and pour over some warmed water or milk. Stir to combine, then add toppings as desired.

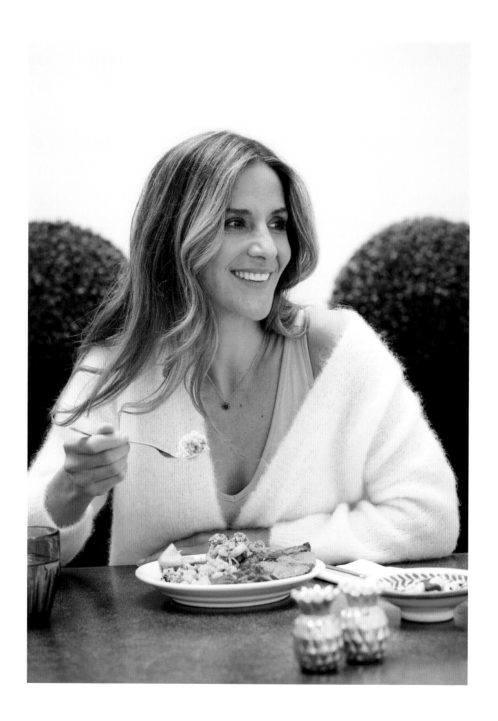

LUNCH

—

Although they say that breakfast is the most important meal of the day, for me it's just one of three very important meals! I believe that every meal is equally important, especially *how* you eat, and *what* you eat. Lunch is the meal that will power you through the afternoon, so that you don't eat highly calorific foods at dinner due to being exhausted.

LUNCH MISTAKES

- Eating 'easy-to-grab' foods that are high in sugar such as a handful of sweets or some biscuits, because you have reached that midday slump.

- Drinking caffeine instead of eating lunch to *'power you through'*. Your slump will only leave you craving highly calorific foods at dinner time.

- Eating at your desk, or while multi-tasking, will not do you any favours. You will most likely not be paying attention and eat excess calories without even noticing.

- Eating on the run is not a good idea either. Your body needs you to eat slowly and digest so that you get the full benefit of your midday fuel stop.

- Not eating enough at lunchtime can spark disastrous dinner effects. Remember, you need more fuel during the day than at night when you are probably just sitting watching TV. So don't skimp on lunch by just getting a green salad. Lunch needs to take you to the finish line, so to speak, and should always have a balance of protein, fat and carbs.

THE BIG LUNCH OFFENDERS

- **PRE-PACKAGED SANDWICHES** – you just don't know how much butter or mayonnaise is packed into your BLT or egg sarnie. If it's a sandwich you want, try to prepare it at home the night before.

- **CAFÉ-/SHOP-BOUGHT SUSHI PACKS** – recent research done on the Channel 4 programme *Food Unwrapped* uncovered that some sushi packs have more more sugar than eight digestive biscuits and more salt than seven packets of crisps! This is because they contain starchy white 'sushi rice' that is mixed with sugary rice vinegar to make it clump together, and the fish and soy sauce also contain high amounts of salt.

⟶ SWITCH TIPS ⟵

- Always try to plan ahead. Using leftovers from last night's dinner is a fantastic way to get ahead of yourself.

- Buy some Tupperware! Packed lunches are not just for kids; all the cool adults are doing it.

- Just as with breakfast, combining carbs, protein and fats at lunchtime will keep your energy reserves topped up. Protein will increase alertness and make you feel full.

- Switch a shop-bought sandwich to a grilled chicken breast with some avocado and brown rice, or a shop-bought sushi pack to some grilled salmon, grilled veg and half a sweet potato with a drizzle of olive oil and a little salt.

- If you are feeling hungry about an hour after lunch, then you might have had a little too much sugar and not enough protein or fat. Have a handful of nuts or some of my DIY trail mix (see page 272) handy if you fall into this trap, so that you can win back your energy without reaching for more sugary pick-me-ups.

QUINOA MÉLANGE

—

- 300g cooked quinoa
  (see quinoa porridge,
  page 227, for cooking
  instructions)
- 1 tsp coconut oil
- 2 stems of purple
  sprouting or tenderstem
  broccoli, chopped
- a handful of green beans,
  chopped
- 1 red pepper, deseeded
  and chopped
- 1 yellow pepper,
  deseeded and chopped
- 1 clove of garlic, peeled
  and chopped
- ½ a thumb-sized piece of
  fresh ginger, peeled and
  grated
- a small handful of cashew
  nuts

**OPTIONAL PROTEIN
SOURCES:**
- chickpeas
- tofu
- grilled salmon or chicken

If you don't have any leftovers in the fridge, cook your quinoa according to the instructions on page 227. Melt the oil in a separate pan and over a medium heat stir-fry the broccoli, green beans, peppers, garlic, ginger and cashew nuts. Once the veg are cooked but still retaining some bite, tip in the quinoa and mix everything together. If you want to increase the protein in this dish, add in some chickpeas or tofu, or grilled salmon or chicken.

SWITCH TIP
This will last in the fridge for a few days and makes for an excellent lunch box on the go.

BYRAM'S BAGUETTE

—

- 1 whole cucumber, peeled and sliced in half lengthways
- 120g grilled chicken or salmon, finely chopped
- some fresh herbs of choice, such as parsley, finely chopped
- 1 tomato, finely chopped
- 1 tbsp black sesame seeds
- 1 tbsp hemp seeds
- a drizzle of olive oil
- a pinch of Himalayan salt

Take a teaspoon and scoop the seeds out of each half of the cucumber (you can add these to smoothies). Mix the chopped chicken or salmon in a bowl with the fresh herbs, tomato, sesame seeds and hemp seeds.

Now fill one cucumber 'trench' with the mixture, drizzle with the oil and sprinkle over the salt. Put the cucumber 'lid' on top and slice. Great served with some toasted dark sourdough or rye on the side.

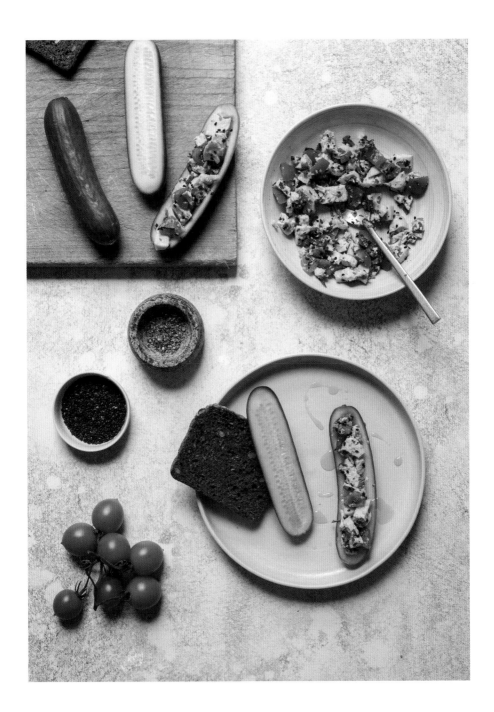

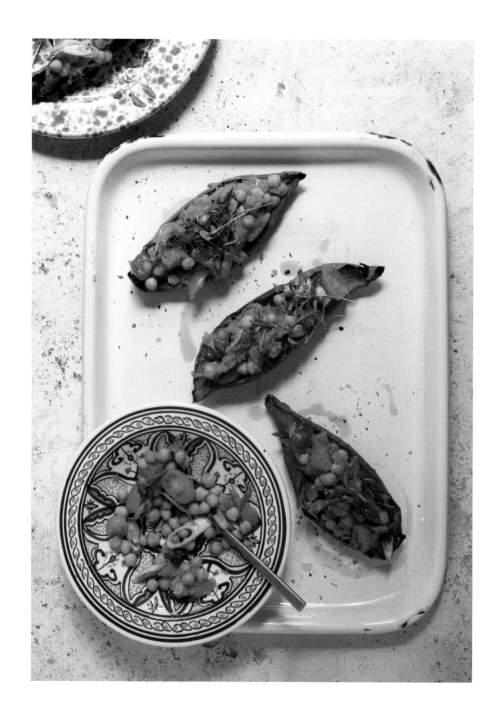

STUFFED SWEET POTATO

—

SERVES 1

- 1 sweet potato, scrubbed
- ½ a 400g tin of chickpeas, drained
- a handful of cherry tomatoes, chopped
- 1 spring onion, finely sliced
- a small handful of fresh basil (optional)
- olive oil

Preheat the oven to 200°C.

Bake the sweet potato until cooked through, which should take about 50 minutes. Slice in half, scoop out the insides and put the contents into a bowl. Leave the empty skin to the side.

Mix the potato insides with the chickpeas, cherry tomatoes, spring onion, basil (if using), and a little olive oil. Pack the mixture back into the potato skins and serve with some grilled chicken or fish.

This is good hot or cold – reheat the stuffing before serving if you'd prefer it hot.

SWITCH TIPS
Switch starchy white potatoes to sweet potatoes when you can – they are chock full of beta-carotene, which is essential for good vision and a healthy immune system. Bake a few sweet potatoes at a time and store them in the fridge to use in other recipes.

BYRAM'S BUMPER BOWL

—

SERVES 2

- 1 sweet potato, sliced
  into wedges
- olive oil
- ground turmeric
- Himalayan salt
- 300g cooked quinoa (see
  page 227) or brown rice
- ½ an avocado, peeled and
  sliced
- 1 carrot, grated
- 1 beetroot, peeled and
  grated
- a couple of handfuls of
  fresh spinach
- black sesame seeds

FOR THE DRESSING:
- 1 tbsp tahini
- 1 tsp honey mustard
- 1 tbsp olive oil
- 1 tsp ground turmeric
- 1 tbsp lime or lemon juice

Preheat the oven to 185°C.

If you don't have leftover quinoa, cook according to the instructions on page 227.

Place the sweet potato wedges on a baking tray lined with parchment, drizzle over some olive oil and sprinkle over some ground turmeric and salt. Roast in the preheated oven for 35–40 minutes (or until cooked).

In the meantime, make the dressing by mixing all the dressing ingredients together in a small bowl or clean jam jar.

Split the cooked quinoa or rice between two bowls and layer over the avocado, grated carrot and beetroot and fresh spinach. Finish with the roasted sweet potato wedges then drizzle the dressing on top. Garnish with a sprinkling of black sesame seeds.

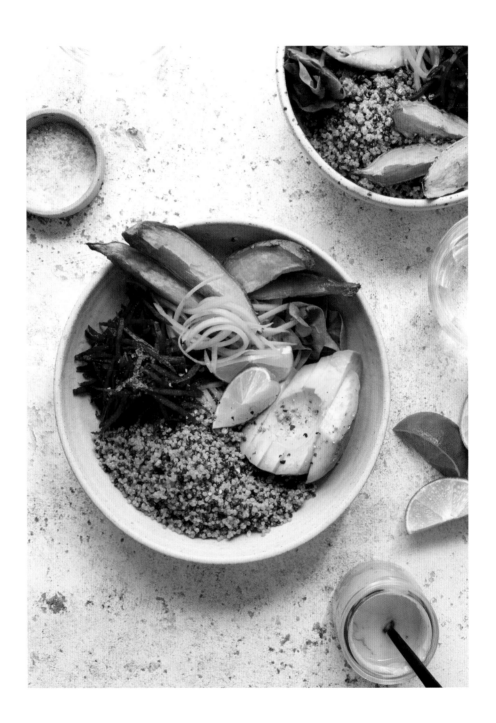

WHITE COURGETTE AND POTATO SOUP

—

SERVES 2 GENEROUSLY

- 2 large courgettes, peeled and chopped
- 1 large potato, peeled and chopped
- 1 litre vegetable stock
- sea salt and freshly ground pepper (optional)

Put the chopped veg in a saucepan and add the vegetable stock. Bring to a boil and simmer for 30 minutes or until the veg are soft. Blend with a stick blender.

Season to taste and serve with some dark bread if desired.

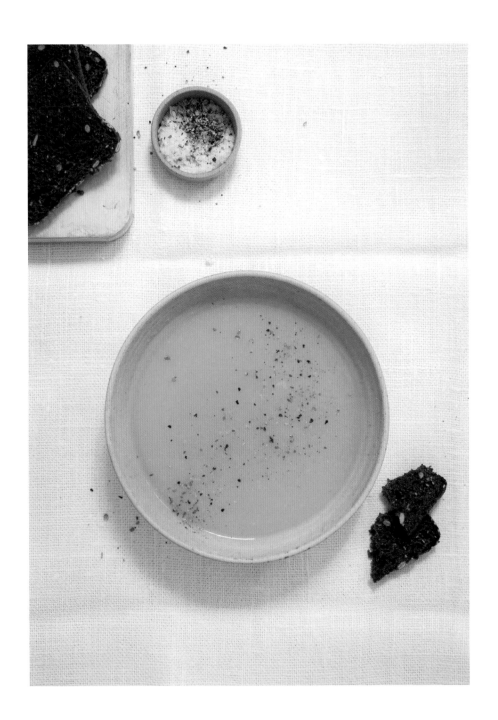

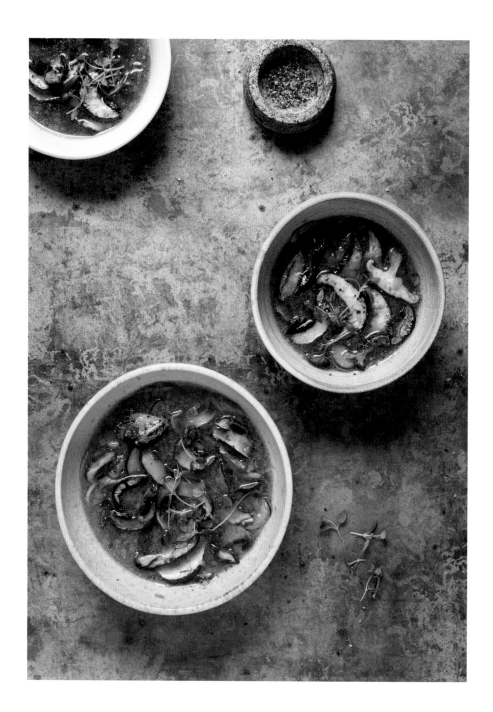

MUSHROOM SOUP

—

SERVES 2

- 2 tbsp rapeseed oil
- 1 small onion, chopped
- 1 clove of garlic, peeled and finely chopped
- 220g mixed mushrooms (chestnut, button and Portobello), chopped
- 1 tsp fresh thyme, leaves picked
- 450ml vegetable stock
- Himalayan salt and freshly ground black pepper

Heat the oil in a medium-sized saucepan. Add in the onion and sauté on a medium heat until translucent, stirring well to make sure it cooks evenly. Turn the heat to low and continue to cook until the onions change colour from white to golden brown and are nicely caramelised. Now add in the garlic, mushrooms and thyme. Cook on a medium heat with the saucepan partially covered for about 10 minutes, until the mushrooms are tender. Add the vegetable stock and bring everything to the boil. Lower the heat and simmer gently, partially covered, for 3–4 minutes.

EASY PEA'SY VEGAN SOUP

—

SERVES 2

- 1 tbsp olive oil
- 1 onion, peeled and chopped
- 3 cloves of garlic, peeled and chopped
- 1 large potato or 2 small, peeled and diced
- 300g peas (fresh or frozen)
- 700ml vegetable broth or water
- Himalayan salt and freshly ground black pepper
- a handful of fresh herbs of choice, such as parsley or thyme, chopped
- 1 tbsp lemon juice

TO SERVE:
- natural vegan yoghurt
- olive oil
- chopped nuts

Heat the oil in a medium-sized pan, add the onion and garlic and fry gently until translucent, stirring occasionally. Add the diced potato and peas, then pour in the vegetable stock/water and season with a pinch of salt and a few grinds of black pepper. Stir through the herbs of your choice and simmer gently on a low heat for 15 minutes, or until the peas and potatoes are soft.

Remove from the heat, add the lemon juice and blend in a blender or in the pot with a stick blender. Divide between two bowls and top with some yoghurt, a drizzle of olive oil and a sprinkle of chopped nuts.

SWITCH TIP
For a heartier meal, you can stir some cooked brown rice or quinoa through the soup. This would make a perfect nutritious dinner.

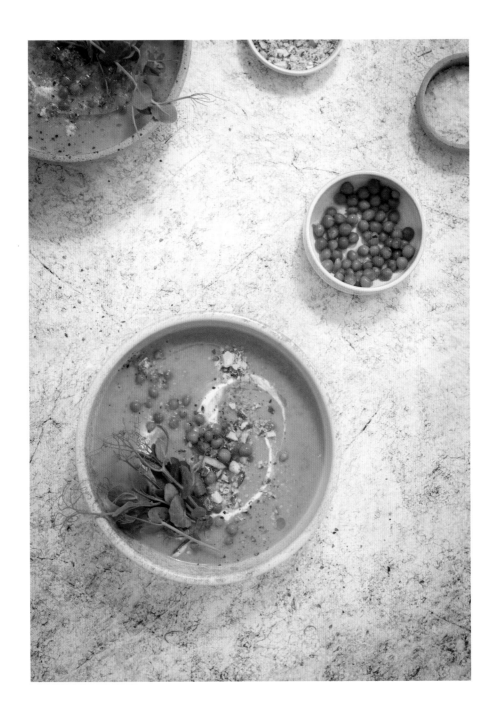

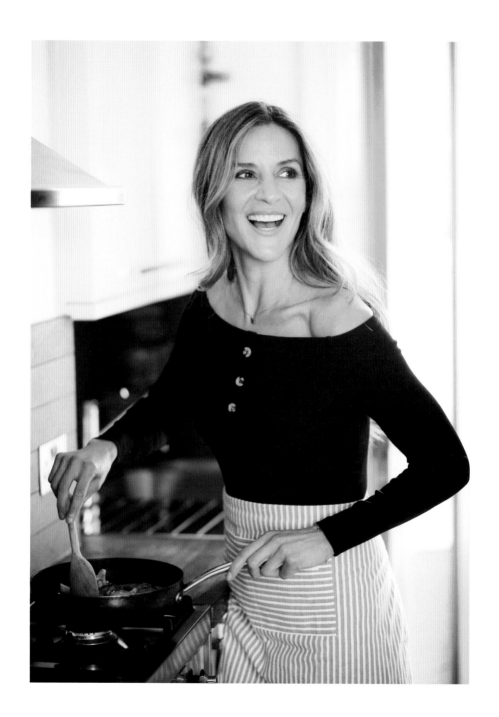

DINNER

—

Dinner can be tough, especially during the working week, because it comes at the end of the day when you're tired or frazzled. And if you've had a really busy or bad day, you might be tempted to throw something together that's not so nutritious, or turn to comfort food such as creamy pasta or cheesy pizza. It's really important to plan this meal properly – if you go to bed malnourished, you won't sleep well.

DINNER MISTAKES

- Bad dinner choices often follow a series of bad choices throughout the day. If you've had an energy-consumptive day or, worse, you haven't fuelled yourself properly throughout the day with a good breakfast and lunch, then dinner will inevitably be an array of bad choices.

- Watching TV while eating dinner is a no-no (although your obsession with *Love Island* might tell you otherwise) because eating in front of the box will stop you eating mindfully and chewing your food. The less you chew, the longer it will take for your food to be digested and therefore you will not feel full, so you will eat more than you need to. And by the time the nutrients get processed, you'll have eaten twice as much as you would have if you had just chewed the first batch properly!

THE BIG DINNER OFFENDERS

- **TAKE-AWAY FOODS** are not considered nutritious meals. They are pumped with cream, salt and sugar and will leave you feeling tired and bloated – ready to fall into bed, yes, but not so ready for a good night's sleep.

- Foods that are **HIGH IN SALT** will not only mess with your sleep-chi but will also make you want to wee-wee. Salty foods will cause sweaty nights, so try to avoid any pre-made foods that are high in sodium.

- Foods such as **WHITE POTATOES**, **WHITE PASTA** and **RICE** or **PIZZA** should be avoided too late in the day. These are foods that are high on the glycaemic index (see page 36), meaning they get absorbed into the bloodstream at a fast rate, giving you a burst of energy, which makes it hard to wind down before bedtime. Also, unless you are a sleepwalking marathon runner, you will not need the energy they provide while you sleep and you might experience sleep disturbances.

⟶ SWITCH TIPS ⟵

- Preparation may be all it takes for you to make a better choice, so always buy ahead and have some lean proteins such as chicken, fish, meat, chickpeas or quinoa on standby. This will stop you being tempted to binge-eat 'comfort' foods.

- Eat earlier. It is important to digest your dinner before you go to bed. So try to eat within a four-hour window of hitting the pillow, otherwise your digestive system will have to go into overdrive while you sleep.

- Avoid eating raw foods, such as salads, in the evening. These take more time for your body to process, at a time when your digestive system should be winding down.

MY GRANNY O'CONNOR'S

TRADITIONAL DUBLIN CODDLE

—

SERVES 6

This recipe is so special to me – I always remember a pot of it boiling away on my Granny's stove when I was a kid. I would run into Granny's house and go straight to the cooker to get a bowl of this scrummy meal. When she passed away, my mum picked up the baton and started making it for us, and then when I was old enough she passed the recipe on to me. It is a typical working-class Dublin dish, made famous for being a meal that you could cook on a tight budget, using up any stray rashers and sausages you had to hand. It brings back so many warm, hearty memories!

- 8 lean butcher's sausages
- 6 good-quality lean bacon rashers
- 1 large onion or 2 small, peeled and sliced
- 2 medium-sized potatoes, peeled and quartered
- bone broth (optional)
- 1 packet of Knorr oxtail soup
- freshly ground black pepper

Place the sausages, bacon, onion and potatoes in a large pot. Season with pepper, pour in enough water and/or bone broth (for a collagen boost) to cover and bring to the boil. Simmer until everything is cooked and the potatoes are soft (about 30 minutes). Now take some of the liquid from the pot, mix with the packet of soup and put back into the pot – this will thicken your coddle. Grind over some pepper if you like –no salt is needed as there will be enough in the bacon and sausages.

SWITCH TIP
As long as they are cooked properly, potatoes are the allies, not the enemies! Not only do they have an extremely high water content (80 per cent), they are also low in fat and calories and are a great source of vitamins and minerals such as potassium and vitamin C. When simply boiled, these Irish friends are a nutritional powerhouse!

HERBED BROWN RICE SERVED WITH SIMPLE POACHED TURKEY BREAST

—

SERVES 2

- 130g brown basmati rice
- 500ml vegetable stock
- 1 bay leaf
- 1 carrot, peeled and chopped
- 1 stick of celery, chopped
- 1 small onion, peeled and chopped
- 2 turkey breasts
- a small handful of fresh parsley, chopped
- a small handful of fresh tarragon, chopped
- a small handful of fresh dill, chopped
- juice of 1 lime
- 1 tbsp linseed or olive oil
- Himalayan salt and freshly ground black pepper

Start by putting your brown rice on to cook according to the instructions on the packet. Brown rice takes longer to cook than white rice, around 45 minutes. While the rice is cooking, you can get on with preparing the poached turkey.

Bring the stock to the boil in a saucepan with the bay leaf, carrot, celery and onion. Add in the turkey, bring to a simmer and cook gently until the turkey is cooked through (around 20 minutes). Remove the turkey from the broth with a slotted spoon and keep warm. You can discard the broth at this point.

When the rice is ready, stir in the herbs, lime juice, oil, salt and pepper. Divide the herbed rice between two plates and put the poached turkey on top.

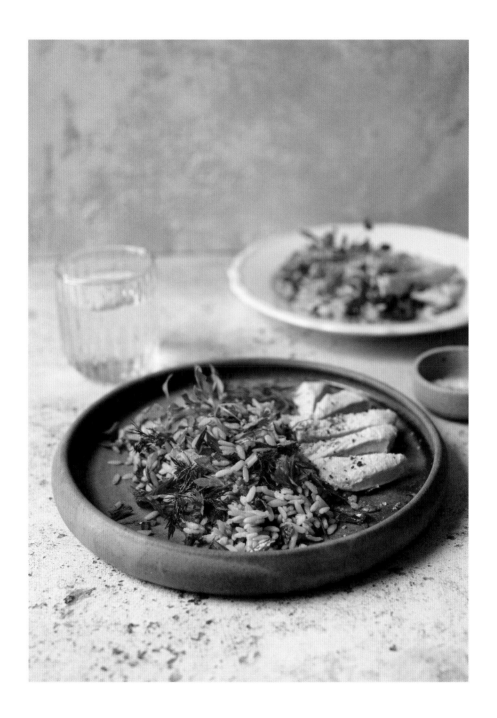

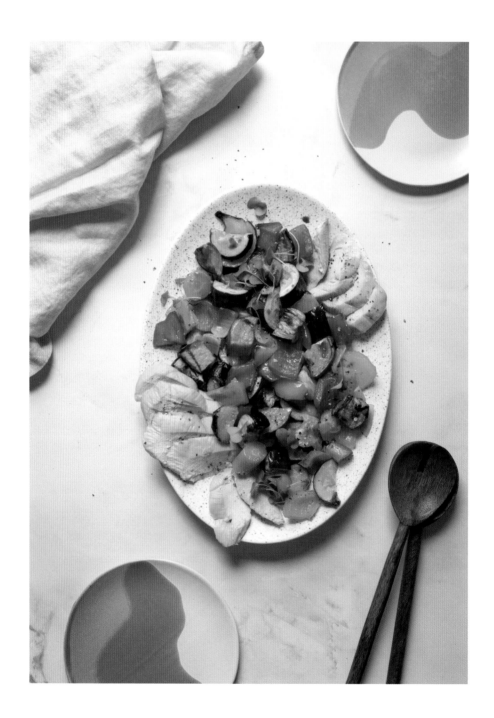

SIMPLE ROASTED VEG

—

SERVES 4

- 2 sweet potatoes, scrubbed and cut into smallish cubes
- 2 onions, peeled and roughly chopped
- 2 carrots, roughly chopped
- 2 courgettes, roughly chopped
- 2 aubergines, roughly chopped
- 1 red pepper, deseeded and roughly chopped
- 1 yellow pepper, deseeded and roughly chopped
- 4 cloves of garlic, peeled
- 1 tbsp olive oil
- 1 tbsp balsamic vinegar

You can add any other veg you have lying around to this dish – these are just suggestions. If you want to use tomatoes, though, add them about 10 minutes after the other veg, as they cook faster.

Preheat the oven to 200°C.

Put all the vegetables in a big bowl, drizzle with the olive oil and sprinkle over some salt. Mix well so everything is well coated. Spread out in a large baking dish lined with baking parchment and place in the preheated oven. Make sure you have the veg in one layer so they cook evenly.

After 20 minutes, remove the dish, toss everything around, and drizzle over the balsamic vinegar. Return to the oven for around 15 minutes, until all the veg are cooked, crispy, and nicely browned.

You can serve these as a side dish with some grilled chicken or fish, or as a main dish on top of a bowl of brown rice.

HEALTHY FISH 'N' CHIPS

—

SERVES 2

- 1 sweet potato, scrubbed and cut into thin wedges
- 2 large parsnips, peeled and cut lengthwise into wedges
- 1 tbsp coconut oil, melted
- 1 tbsp coconut flour
- sea salt
- a generous handful of mixed thyme, basil and rosemary, finely chopped
- 75g almonds, finely chopped
- 1 tbsp olive oil
- pinch of sea salt
- 2 fillets sustainably sourced white fish – I use sea bass or cod

Preheat the oven to 180°C.

Arrange the sweet potato and parsnip wedges on a large, parchment-lined baking sheet. Drizzle over the coconut oil and sprinkle with the coconut flour and a pinch of sea salt. Place in the oven and roast for 25 minutes.

Meanwhile, prepare your herb-nut crust. Put the herbs and almonds in a bowl and mix in the olive oil and a pinch of sea salt. This mixture should be quite well bound, so add more oil if it's not sticking together enough. Slather the mixture over the fish fillets so they are completely covered.

Remove the baking tray of veg 'chips', and move to one side to make room for the fish. Place the crusted fish on the tray and return to the oven until the fish is cooked through (about 20 minutes more).

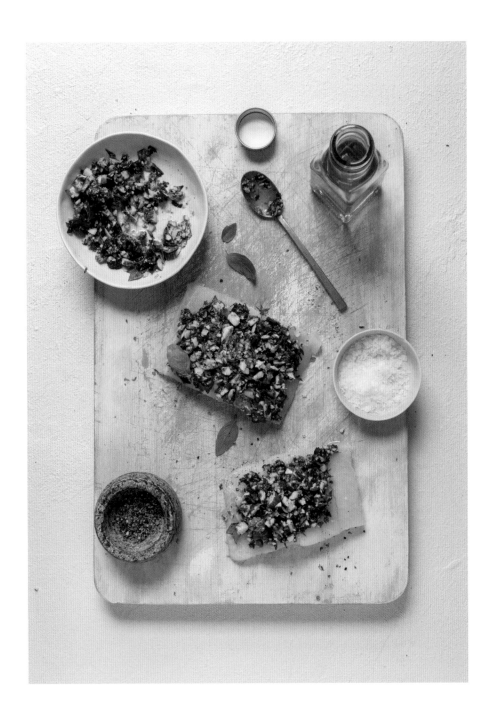

MY GRANNY PERIN'S HEALTHY CURRY

—

SERVES 4

Not all curries have to be unhealthy. My dad's mum, Granny Perin, was Persian and everything she cooked was from scratch, using only fresh, organic ingredients. She passed on her divine curry recipe to my dad; it's simple, tasty and the real deal.

- 2 tbsp ghee, coconut oil or rapeseed oil
- ½ an onion, peeled and finely sliced
- 2 cloves of garlic, peeled and chopped
- ½ a thumb-sized piece of fresh ginger, peeled and finely chopped
- 4 tsp curry spice powder (shop-bought or homemade – see below)
- 400g protein of choice – tofu, fish, chicken or meat, chopped
- 3 tbsp tomato purée
- 1–2 400g tins of tomatoes (2 if you want more sauce)
- 1 stock cube
- 1 tbsp natural yoghurt (optional)

CURRY POWDER:
- ½ tsp chilli power
- 1 tsp ground coriander
- 1 tsp curry powder
- 1 tsp garam masala
- 1 tsp ground cumin
- ¼ tsp ground turmeric

If you are making your own curry powder, simply mix all the ingredients together in a small bowl: if you like, double the quantities and store in a clean jar to use again.

In a large pan, fry the onion slices in the oil until light golden. Add the garlic and ginger followed by the curry spices, adding a little water to stop them burning and stirring constantly to make sure they don't stick. Do this for approximately 1 minute to 'cook' the spices, but be careful not to let them burn.

If using chicken or meat, add at this stage and fry, stirring well to coat in the spices. When the protein is starting to take on some colour, add the tomato purée and tin(s) of tomatoes, then sprinkle in the stock cube. If you are using fish or tofu for your protein, add this now; it takes less time to cook. Simmer the curry gently for about 15 minutes more until cooked through and fragrant. Swirl through some natural yoghurt before serving, if you like.

Serve with basmati rice or naan bread.

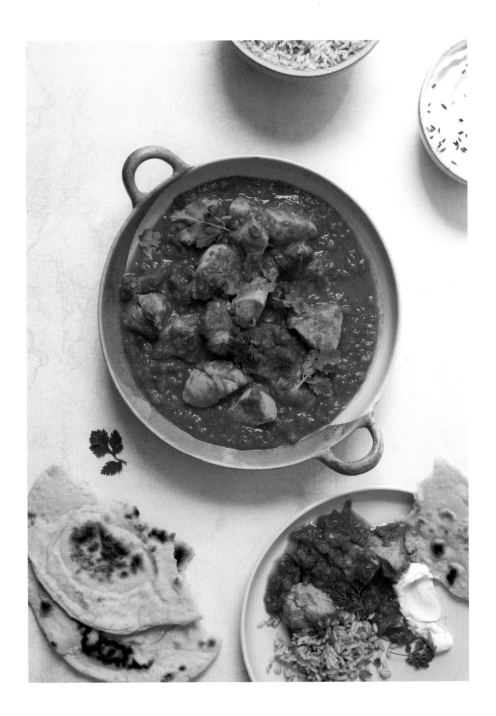

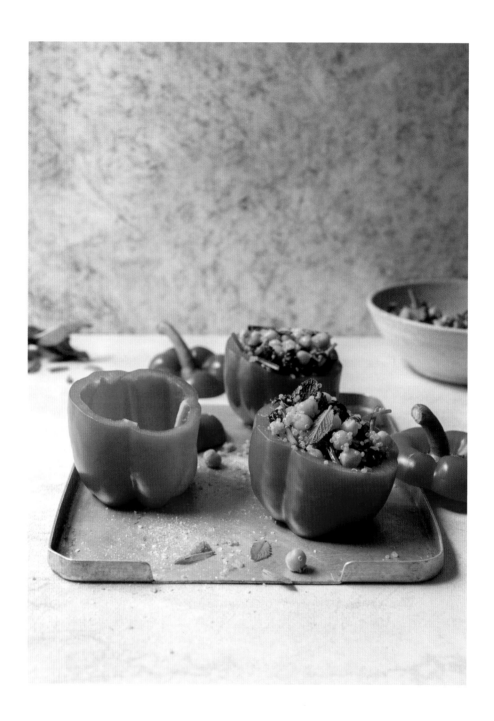

STUFFED PEPPERS

—

- 1 tbsp coconut oil
- 1 clove of garlic, chopped
- a sprinkle of chilli powder
- ½ a thumb-sized piece of fresh ginger, peeled and grated
- 1 x 400g tin of chickpeas, drained
- a couple of handfuls of fresh spinach
- 300g cooked quinoa (see quinoa porridge, page 227, for cooking instructions)
- a sprig of fresh mint, leaves chopped
- 4 red peppers, tops removed and seeds scooped out

Preheat the oven to 180°C.

If you don't have any leftover quinoa, prepare as per the instructions on page 227.

Heat the oil in a medium-sized pan and stir-fry the garlic, chilli and ginger until softened. Add in the chickpeas, then the spinach. When the spinach is wilted, stir in the cooked quinoa and the fresh mint.

Carefully fill each pepper with this mixture, then place on a baking sheet lined with parchment. Cook in the preheated oven for about 25 minutes until the peppers are softened and the filling is cooked.

BYRAM'S TURKEY BURGER

—

SERVES 2

- 200g turkey mince
- juice of 2 limes
- 1 spring onion, finely chopped
- sea salt and freshly ground black pepper
- olive oil, for frying
- ½ an avocado, smashed
- 2 tomatoes, sliced
- ½ a red onion, peeled and finely sliced
- 2 brown buns – dark buckwheat rolls if available

In a bowl, mix the turkey mince, lime juice, spring onion, salt and pepper. Let the mixture sit in the fridge for 30 minutes to marinate.

Now it's time to make the burgers. With clean hands, shape the turkey mix into two patties. Lightly fry in a little olive oil until golden brown on both sides and cooked through.

Assemble your burgers: get your rolls and spread the smashed avocado on half of each, followed by the slices of tomato and onion. Pop your burger on top and finish with the other half of the roll.

Serve with a few wedges of simple sweet potato fries or some simple roasted vegetables (see page 251).

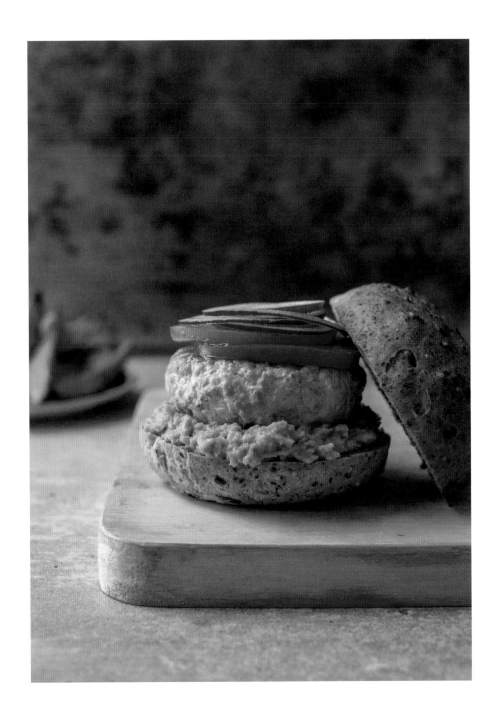

SUPER SNACKS

—

I love snacks! Some experts don't agree with snacking, insisting that you should only have three square meals a day. But like many of us, I feel dips in energy in between the big three, therefore my motto is: 'if you must snack, snack wisely'!

SNACK MISTAKES

- Don't snack out of boredom or stress. If you feel you're about to do this, drink a glass of fizzy water with a squeeze of lemon instead.

- Make sure to snack mindfully, not mindlessly. For example, snacking on a bag of salt and vinegar crisps while watching *Keeping Up with the Kardashians* is mindless. Chopping up an apple, taking a scoop of peanut butter, spreading it on thinly, and thoroughly chewing and tasting it, is mindful.

- Do not snack too often on foods that are high in sugar, salt or trans fats (see page 39). Foods with protein will keep you fuller for longer, and foods with good carbs will help you to carry on tasks for longer.

- Plan ahead. Make sure you always have a supply of things you can grab and put in your bag, such as sliced vegetables with hummus dips (see my DIY spreads, page 265) or pre-make bags of trail mix (see page 272).

- Pay attention to portion sizes when snacking. Snacks are not meals, just an in-between. So perhaps have the fridge stocked with small Tupperware boxes of snacks about the size of your palm.

THE BIG SNACK OFFENDERS

- **CRACKERS AND CRISPS** are seemingly easy snacks, yet they will leave you craving more due to the salt content, which in turn will leave you dehydrated.

- While **NUTS** are a fantastic snack, it's important not to consume too many. A large handful can often contain 500 calories or more – sometimes the same calorie content as a full meal. Try not to fall into the trap of eating more than approximately 10 nuts in one sitting.

- **CEREAL BARS** are often packed with sugar, so be mindful if you choose these as a snack choice. These will not keep you full for long, especially if they have a high sugar content. Switch these for pre-made bags of trail mix with nuts, seeds and some cacao nibs and dried berries (see page 272).

- **FLAVOURED YOGHURTS** are a no-no when it comes to snacking, because not only are they packed with sugar, they also contain a lot of artificial flavourings and colourings.

→ SWITCH TIPS ←

- Switch sugary milk chocolate for dark chocolate or cacao. The darker the chocolate, the better it is for you.

- Switch biscuits for rice cakes, corn cakes or oatcakes. Have these with some avocado because it's not too heavy but is still a good carb injection – the good fats in avocado will keep your blood sugar stable all day. They don't call avocado 'God's butter' for no reason!

- Switch the Creme Egg for a boiled egg! This may sound random, but I sometimes carry hard-boiled eggs with me as a healthy snack. They are a great source of protein and fat and therefore can see you through moments of hunger and will stop you snacking on sugary treats.

BYRAM'S BANANA SPLIT

—

SERVES 1

- 1 banana, peeled and sliced in half lengthways
- 1 tbsp nut butter of choice
- 1 tbsp Greek/vegan yoghurt
- a sprinkle of ground cinnamon
- 1 tsp black sesame seeds

Spread the nut butter on one side of the sliced banana, and the Greek/vegan yoghurt on the other half. Sandwich the banana back together again. Sprinkle some cinnamon and sesame seeds on top. Cut into diagonal slices and enjoy!

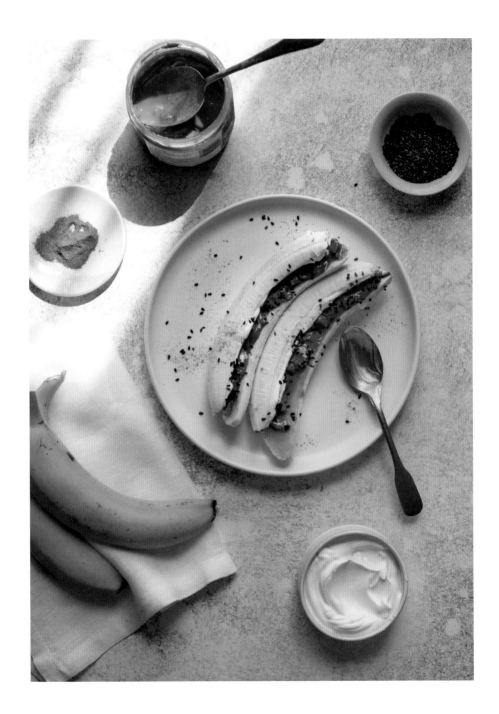

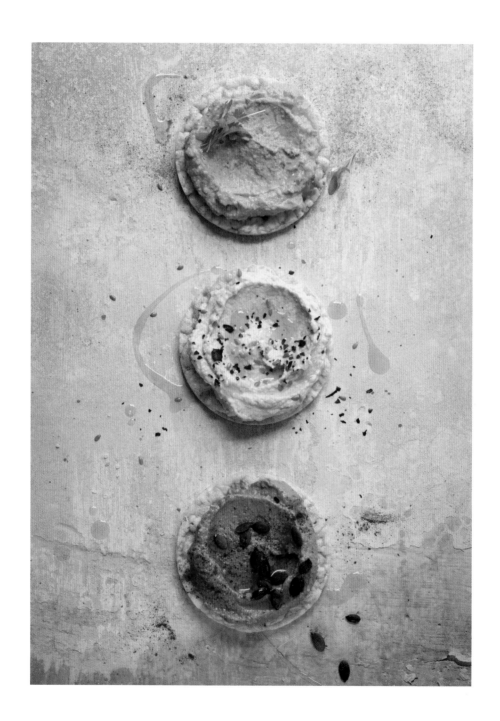

EASY DIY SPREADS

—

Spreads are the perfect accompaniment to snack on with crudités or on oat, rice or corn cakes. Here are some of my favourite options – all easy to make and delicious!

PLAIN HUMMUS

– 1 x 400g tin of chickpeas
– 4 tbsp olive oil
– 4 tbsp water
– 1 tbsp tahini
– 1 tsp black sesame seeds
– a small amount of garlic (to personal taste)
– juice of one lemon
– salt to taste

Simply blend all the ingredients together.

SWEET POTATO HUMMUS

– 2 sweet potatoes
– 4 tbsp olive oil
– salt, to taste

Peel then boil the sweet potatoes, or roast them in their jackets at 200°C until soft. Blend the flesh with 4 tbsp olive oil and salt to taste.

BEETROOT HUMMUS

– 1 large beetroot
– ½ a 400g tin of chickpeas
– the juice of a ½ a lemon
– 2 tbsp olive oil
– salt, to taste

Peel and roast the beetroot, wrapped in foil, at 200°C until soft. Put in a blender with the rest of the ingredients and blend until smooth.

AVOCADO AND LEMON MASH

– 1 avocado
– juice of half a lemon
– a pinch of Himalayan salt

Simply scoop the flesh of an avocado into a bowl with the lemon juice and salt. Mash with a fork until smooth.

ORANGE ALMOND BUTTER SPREAD

– 4 large carrots, peeled and chopped
– 3 tsp almond butter

Steam the carrots for 25–30 minutes until soft. Add the almond butter and blend.

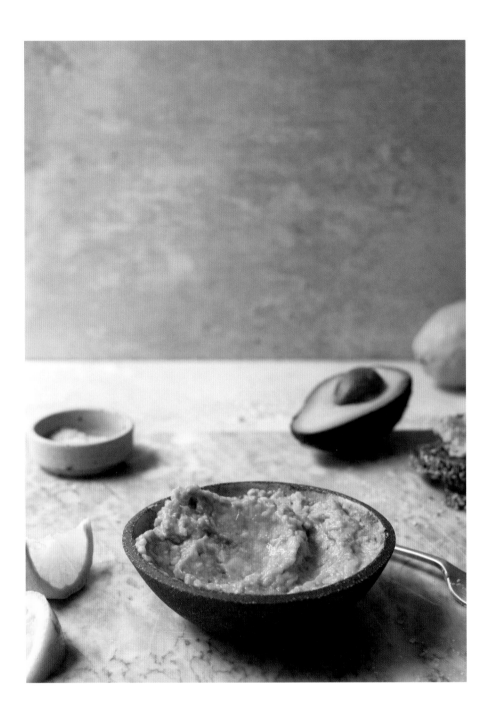

DIY JAM

- a punnet of berries
- juice of half a lemon
- ½ a thumb of fresh
  ginger, peeled
  and grated
- 1 tsp vanilla extract
- 3 tbsp chia seeds

Cook the punnet of berries in a small saucepan over a medium heat and smash them up into a pulp. Add the lemon juice, ginger and vanilla extract. Remove from the heat and allow to cool, then stir through the chia seeds and allow to settle.

Decant into a jam jar and store in the fridge for up to a week. Try it dolloped on top of your oatmeal or spread on toast.

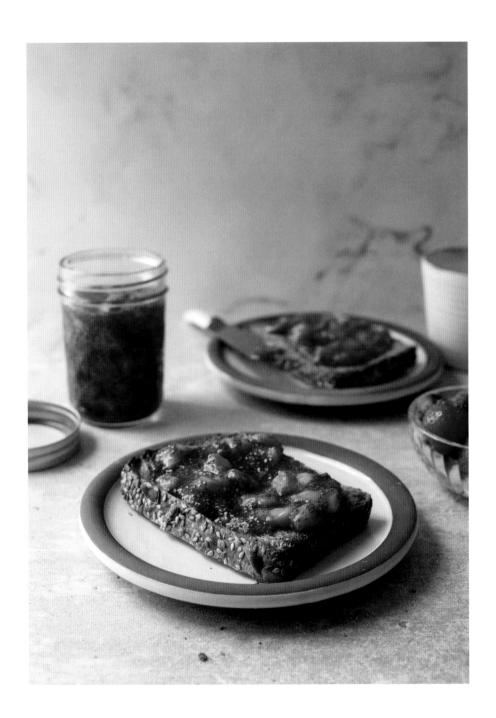

TURMERIC KALE CHIPS

—

SERVES 2

- a bag of kale (about 200g), washed, woody stalks removed, leaves torn into bite-sized pieces
- a drizzle of olive oil
- a pinch of Himalayan salt
- a pinch of ground turmeric

Preheat the oven to 150°C.

Put the kale in a large bowl and drizzle over some olive oil and salt. With clean hands, 'massage' the salt into the kale for about 5 minutes – this will tenderise it. Add some turmeric for an extra kick.

Arrange the kale in a single layer on one or two roasting trays lined with baking parchment and place in the oven until crisp (about 20 minutes).

SWITCH TIP
These are a perfect snacking alternative to greasy chips or crisps.

SWEET CORN CAKES

—

SERVES 1

- 2 corn cakes
- thick Greek/vegan yoghurt
- a handful of fresh blueberries
- a pinch of ground cinnamon
- a sprinkle of coconut flakes

Simply spread the yoghurt on to the corn cake then add the blueberries, cinnamon and coconut flakes. Enjoy!

DIY TRAIL MIX

—

- 2 handfuls of cacao nibs
- 2 handfuls of seeds and nuts of choice
- 2 handfuls of dried mulberries or goji berries
- 2 handfuls of coconut flakes

Mix everything together and store in a Tupperware box. Then put one handful into a Ziploc bag every morning, and take it with you to nibble on through the day.

APPLE AND NUT BUTTER

—

- 1 apple, sliced
- 2 tbsp nut butter of choice

Pop the sliced apple into a Tupperware box and the nut butter into another smaller box. When ready to snack, simply spread some nut butter onto each slice of apple and enjoy!

SWITCH TIP
Snack on this when you're tired. The fat in the nut butter will slow the rate at which the sugar in the apple hits your bloodstream.

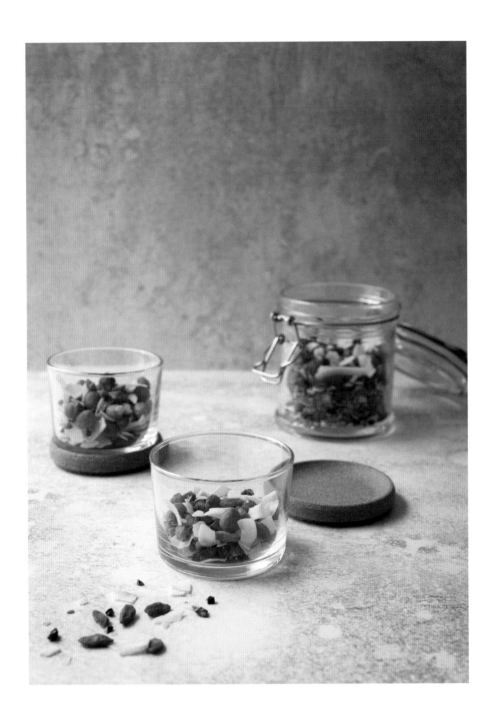

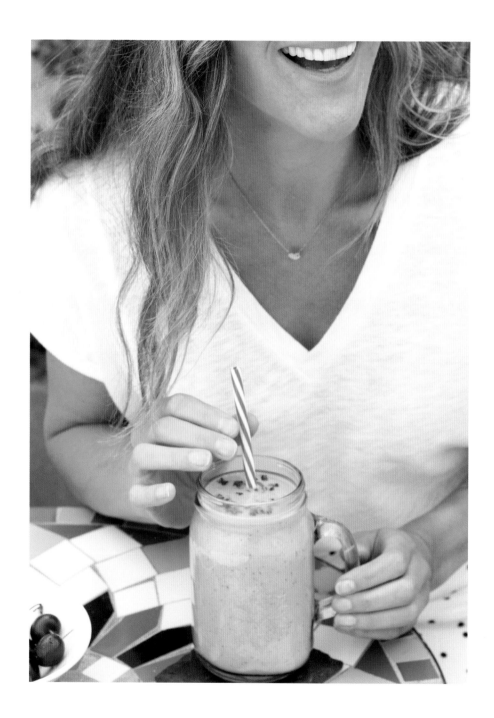

DESSERTS AND SMOOTHIES

—

For many years, I denied myself desserts and all that happened was that I craved sweet treats even more, which led to a binge-purge-repeat cycle. It took me a long time to understand that it is important to treat yourself, and desserts are a perfectly acceptable addition to your daily intake – just as long as you eat them like any other meal: in moderation, eating only what you need to satisfy that sweet tooth. So over the years I sought out alternatives and learned how to twist classic high-calorie, sugar-laden desserts into my own healthy versions. These recipes still pack an indulgent punch and will satisfy any sweet cravings you might have.

Smoothies are an extremely simple way to get a nutritious and filling snack, breakfast blast or, depending on the ingredients, a speedy lunch. You can load them with a range of fibrous vegetables, fruits, superfoods, protein (powders) and even grains (such as oats), so don't pass them off as just a simple drink – they pack a real punch when it comes to nutrition.

MORNING POWER GREEN MACHINE

—

SERVES 1–2

- 120ml almond milk or coconut water
- 120ml filtered water
- ½ a peeled banana, frozen
- 1 kiwi, peeled
- a big handful of baby spinach leaves
- a thumb-sized piece of fresh ginger
- 4–5 ice cubes
- 1 teaspoon of matcha green tea powder

Blitz all the ingredients together in a blender.

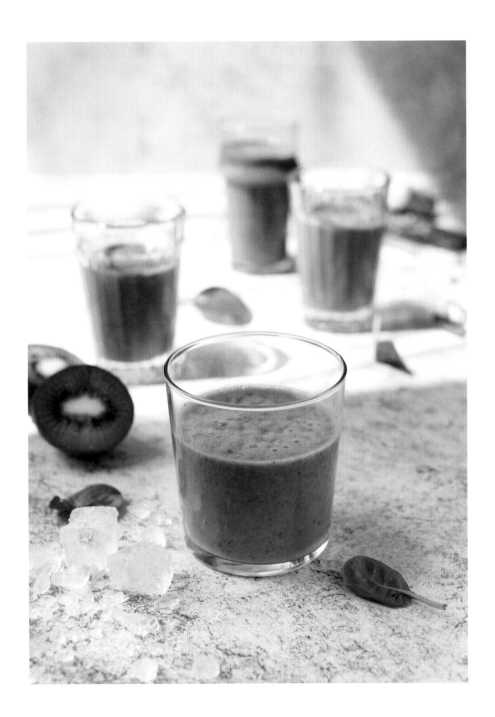

PROTEIN POWER BREAKFAST SMOOTHIE

—

SERVES 1

- 500ml almond milk
- 1 scoop vegan protein powder
- 45g gluten-free oats
- ¼ avocado
- a handful of fresh spinach/2 cubes of frozen spinach
- a handful of berries or ½ an apple
- a pinch of ground cinnamon

OPTIONAL ADDITIONS:
- ½ a banana, peeled (for extra sweetness/ thickness)
- 1 tsp agave syrup (optional for extra sweetness)
- 1 tsp maca powder
- 2 tbsp flax seeds
- 2 tsp chia seeds (an excellent source of omega-3 and they make the smoothie thicker)

Whizz everything together in a blender and serve in a tall glass. Perfect for a sustaining breakfast on the go!

SUPERWOMAN PROTEIN SHAKE

—

SERVES 1–2

- ½ a banana
- ½ an avocado
- 2 dates, pitted
- 1 tsp spirulina powder
- 2 tsp almond butter
- 1 scoop vegan/whey
  protein powder
- 400ml soya or nut milk
- 1 cup coconut water
- a handful of fresh
  spinach leaves

Whizz everything together in a blender.

SWITCH TIP
This is a great post-workout recovery smoothie.

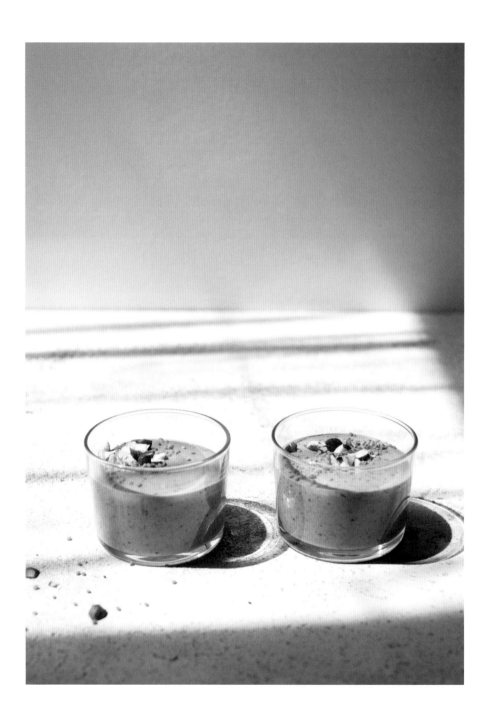

SUPERFOOD SMOOTHIE

—

SERVES 1–2

- ½ a banana
- ¼ mango (optional)
- 2 tsp chia seeds
- 1 tsp maca powder
- 1 tbsp goji berries
- 1 tsp bee pollen
- 1 tbsp hemp seeds
- 500ml almond milk
- a handful of blueberries

TOPPING:
- a handful of crushed nuts
  and dried mulberries

Blitz all the ingredients together in a blender and top with the nuts and mulberries.

CHOCOLATE PROTEIN SMOOTHIE BOWL

—

SERVES 1

- a scoop of chocolate
  protein powder
- ½ an avocado
- 45g gluten-free oats
- a handful of berries (I
  use blueberries)
- 2 tablespoon chia seeds
- a pinch of ground
  cinnamon (optional)
- 500ml water or nut milk
- 2 ice cubes

TOPPING:
- 2 tbsp cacao nibs
- 2 tbsp goji berries
- coconut flakes

Blitz the smoothie ingredients in a blender until smooth. Once blended and thick, pour into a bowl. Sprinkle the cacao nibs, goji berries and coconut flakes on top.

SWITCH TIP
Sometimes my smoothies (like this one) are so thick that I pour them into a bowl and eat them with a spoon – that way it feels as though I am eating them as a meal! It's amazing how a simple mindset switch like this can make a difference.

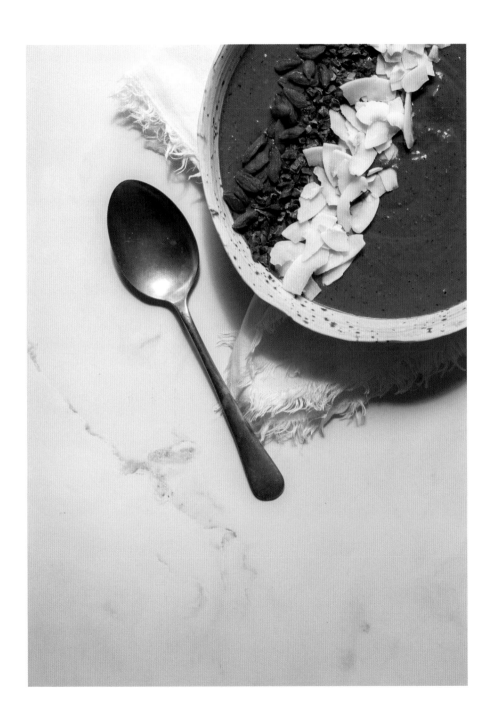

GLOWING GREEN SMOOTHIE

—

SERVES 1–2

- a handful of kale, washed
- a handful of baby
  spinach, washed
- ½ a cucumber, sliced
- ¼ avocado
- juice of ½ a lemon
- 1 banana, peeled
- ½ a thumb-sized piece of
  fresh ginger
- 200ml coconut water
- 200ml water
- a few ice cubes

Put all the ingredients into a blender and blend until smooth and creamy. Add ice depending on your temperature preference.

SWITCH TIPS

- Frozen bananas can work well in smoothies as they have the added bonus of making them nice and cold without adding ice. Simply peel, slice into chunks and place in a large Ziploc bag in the freezer to use when needed.

- Add more spinach and kale to increase nutritional benefits.

BEN'S BROWNIES

—

MAKES 10–15 BROWNIES

It took me years to find alternative healthy ingredients and methods to make one of my favourite desserts – the chocolate fudge brownie. I just couldn't quite figure out what to add that would still have the same famous melt-in-your-mouth texture that a fudge brownie has … until my good friend and vegan chef Ben Whale created these beauties!

- 150ml water
- 2 tbsp milled flax seeds
- 2 tbsp almond butter
- 2 tbsp coconut oil
- 350g dates, stoned
- 100g cacao powder
- 1 tsp vanilla extract
- 180g aduki beans, cooked

Preheat the oven to 150°C and line a 23cm square baking tin with parchment.

Mix the water and the milled flax seeds together to make a thick, gelatinous egg replacement. Then put the almond butter, coconut oil, flax 'egg' and dates in a food processor and blend until smooth. Add in the cacao powder, vanilla and aduki beans and blend again until smooth. Pour the batter into the prepared tin and bake for 20 minutes until crusty on top. Remove from the oven and allow to cool, then cut into squares.

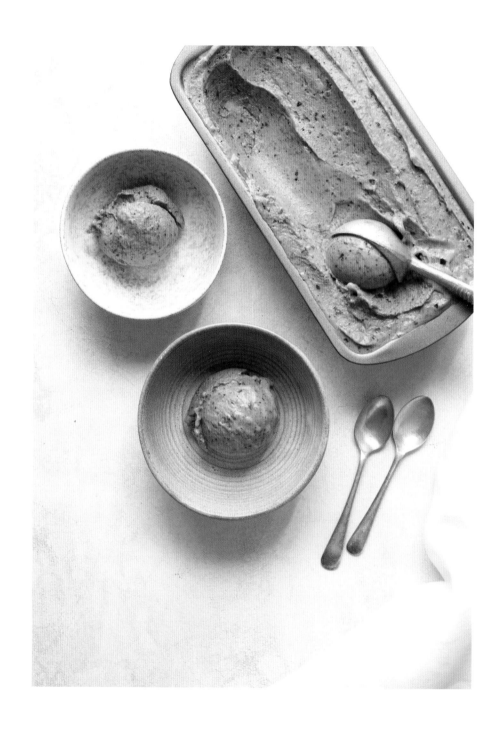

GOJI BERRY AND OATMEAL BISCUITS

—

MAKES 15 BISCUITS

- 120g goji berries
- 160g wholewheat flour
- 2 tsp baking powder
- 1 tsp ground cinnamon
- 65g oats
- 2 tbsp coconut oil
- 170ml agave syrup
- 3 egg whites
- 2 tsp vanilla extract

Preheat the oven to 170°C.

Soak the goji berries in water for about 10 minutes until soft, drain, then squeeze out all excess water. Combine all your dry ingredients in one bowl. Mix the wet ingredients in another bowl, then add this mix to the dry and stir well. Spoon about 15 rounds on to a baking sheet lined with parchment, making sure to leave some space between the biscuits so they can expand. Bake in the preheated oven for about 15 minutes, until golden. Remove from the oven and allow to cool. Store in an airtight container in the fridge for up to a week or in the freezer for up to 6 months.

HEALTHY BANANA-BERRY ICE CREAM

—

SERVES 2–4

I scream you scream we all scream for ice cream! Who doesn't love sitting down with a tub of the cold stuff and a big spoon? This recipe is low in fat, but high in natural sugars, so go easy on your portions. It yields about three cups, so one cup will be plenty for a sweet treat.

- 2 peeled, frozen bananas, sliced (make sure you slice before you freeze)
- 1 cup (130g) frozen berries of choice
- 2 tbsp agave syrup
- ½ cup coconut or almond milk

Put all the ingredients into a food processor and blend until creamy. This process takes a few minutes and you may need to be patient and stop and stir a few times. Store in the freezer in a Tupperware container (if it doesn't all get eaten in the first sitting).

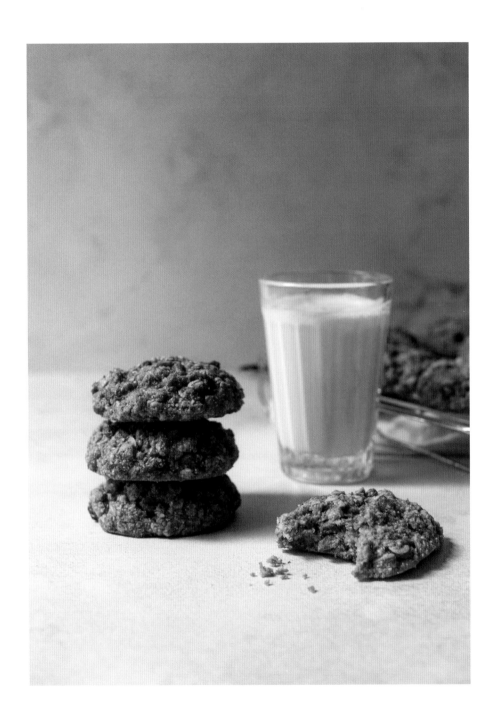

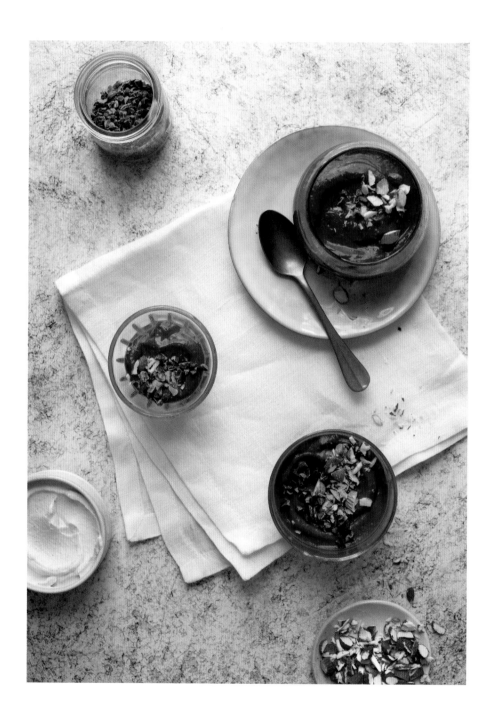

HEALTHY CHOCOLATE MOUSSE

—

SERVES 1

- 1 avocado
- 2 tbsp cacao powder
- 2 tbsp maple syrup
- a sprinkle of nuts and cacao nibs

Blend the first three ingredients together until mousse-like in consistency. Serve with sprinkles of nuts and cacao nibs.

LET'S DATE!

—

SERVES 2

- 6 tsp nut butter
- 6 dates, pitted

Put a teaspoon of nut butter inside each date, and pop in the freezer. Great as a snack or dessert.

AND FINALLY ...

Ladies ... now I must leave you to go forth and conquer. Never forget that continuous improvement is better than delayed perfection, so I urge you to go slowly, be kind to yourselves, and let the seeds of knowledge I have shared with you grow with care. Don't waste another day waiting for life to happen, when you can make The Switch right now!

ACKNOWLEDGEMENTS

Ah, the section that I am most excited about – this is where I get to express my gratitude! I would like to use this as an opportunity to practise what I preach and write my daily gratitude journal.

I am grateful for my husband Julian, who has championed me and lifted me up every day since we met. Julian, during the process of writing this book, you saved me from a few 'funky' situations. Thank you for pouring your heart and soul into this book as much as I did, for taking the time to understand my words and my thoughts, and in turn giving me the confidence to put them on paper. Thank you for always expressing your pride in me and for being by my side to remind and reassure me that 'I got this'!

I am grateful for my family, in particular my parents Betty and Denny, my original champions, who have always been proud of me no matter what. Thank you, Mum and Dad, for teaching me to chase my dreams and instilling in me that no dream was too big or too far-fetched. Thank you for encouraging me to always do what makes me happy and to eliminate things in my life that do not serve me. Thank you for teaching me early lessons in switching the narrative! And I am grateful for my big sis Natasha, who has always taken her little sister's hand and guided her through life with wisdom, pragmatism and love.

I am grateful to the wonderful team at Gill Books. Thank you to Sarah, Catherine, Teresa and all the team for believing in me to write this book. Thank you for putting your faith in me as a first-time author, and for being my first publisher. Thank you for getting this book made, despite the many barriers we all encountered with COVID-19.

I am grateful to all of the women who have come to me for advice over the years and who have told me my words helped them. To you I am grateful for giving me the courage to write this book. I thank you for heeding my words on how to stop the cycle of destructive dieting and the constant need to be perfect. I was heartened by your successes, and these successes encouraged me to distil a lifetime of my experiences, knockdowns and bounce-backs into the form of this book.

I am grateful to the universe, which always has my back, because no matter what happens in life, whether we are thriving or just surviving, the time will be right when the universe says it's time. Thank you, universe, for giving me an assignment, and for showing me where to go and what to do.

And I am grateful to YOU, whoever you are, reading these words right now. Yes, YOU. Thank you from the bottom of my heart for putting your faith in me to pick up this book and read it; you will never know how much that means to me. I am sending you the strength to carry out the actions that I know you have within you to make The Switch.

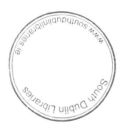